12STEPS
to OPTIMAL
WELL-BEING

"Add more life to your years"

KRUTI THAKORE

12 Steps to Optimal Well-Being

"Add more life to your years"

My vision is to see a healthy world by creating awareness and inspiring people to make easily sustainable lifestyle changes. This book will empower you with a healthy mindset and knowledge to achieve optimal well-being by creating a simplified, easy-to-follow, personalized holistic daily routine.

If you would like support in staying motivated throughout your well-being journey, email me at inquiries@krutithakore.com.

Disclaimer

The information in this book contains the opinions and ideas of its author. It is intended to provide helpful and informative material on the subjects addressed in the book. It is published with an understanding that the author and the publisher are not engaged in rendering medical services. The reader should consult their medical, health, or other competent professional before drawing inferences from it. The author and publisher expressly disclaim all responsibility for any liability, loss, or risk, personal or otherwise, that is incurred as a consequence, directly or indirectly, of the use and application of any of the book's contents.

In case you choose to use any of the information from the book for yourself, the author assumes no responsibility for your actions, and is not liable for any personal injury, including death, caused by your use or misuse of the book or the author's website and its content.

The author has used her best efforts in preparing this book, and every attempt has been made to source all the information from credible resources; the sources of the data have been given due credit.

As we know well, knowledge is power! Kruti has an ocean of knowledge in the health and wellness field, and through this book, she has made it accessible to everyone in easy-to-understand simple steps. After reading this book, I came away with deep respect for the human body and its intricacies and the tools that Kruti has provided to help keep the body, mind, and spirit in the best of shape. She has combined the age-old wisdom of Eastern Ayurvedic medicine with Western advances in the field and brought us the best steps for optimal health. Reading your book has made me realize that optimal health is achievable for everyone!

Arti Khare
Partner and Vice President, Caresoft Inc.

Finally, a self-help book that's not just about achieving goals through positive thinking. The state of complete well-being is the art of aligning mind, body, and spirit, and the author explains why certain factors must be present. She imparts knowledge of all these dimensions with clarity of thought and easy-to-follow guidelines. Kruti loves and cares deeply for her family, friends, and all around her, and this is evident in her passion to help everyone live an optimal lifestyle.

Tamminay Otoo
CEO, Arabees Wellness

As a busy professional working 50 plus hours a week, I always felt that I hardly had time to focus on my health and well-being. It felt like I was compromising on my health while focusing on my career, but after reading this book, I realized that optimal well-being is not rocket science. As a scientist, I have always been drawn to evidence-based practices. 12 Steps to Optimal Well-Being taught me to leverage little cracks of my nonproductive time to improve my well-being so that I can be more productive in my professional and personal life.

A.T.

Sr. Research Scientist

I love this book. I like how the author has put together science along with ancient concepts that help to promote a healthy lifestyle. The definitions of how our body functions were impressive. I've long had questions about vitamins and how certain foods affect our body and mind, which this book answers. If you have ever wondered about Ayurvedic medicine, the impact of what you consume, and have always wanted a step-by-step guide on positive health habits, then this book is that guide. 12 Steps to Optimal Well-Being is an impressive read and extensively researched. I'm so glad I was able to be one of the first readers of this book.

Linda Quick,

Broker Associate - The Quick Response Team
Circle Of Excellence 2007, 2009-2021
RE/MAX Platinum Club Member - top 9% of Agents Nationwide
Re/Max Select

Thank You

First and foremost, the glory goes to God. My special thanks to my parents for giving me life, education, the right values, and nurturing so that I can shine my light every day. I am blessed to have a supportive husband and son who have loved, motivated, and supported me in my journey of writing and publishing this book. Also, I am very thankful to The Chopra Center, YogaMedCo, and Cornell University, for the knowledge I have received in nutrition, healthy living, integrative health, health and wellness coaching, and Ayurveda. I still have a lot to learn, and I strive for excellence every day. I aspire to continue my journey in this field.

I am blessed to have support from my mentors, friends, and family members, who love me, support me, and have stood by me through thick and thin. Also, I am thankful to Dr. Suzie Carmack of YogaMedCo for the guidance and support throughout the publishing journey. I am grateful to have you all as my strong backbone and support system in my life.

Last but not least, this book would not have been published and reached all the readers without the support of the crew that worked behind the scenes to make my vision a reality. I am grateful for their contribution and support. Also, my special thanks to the readers of this book for their love and support.

Namaste!

Contents

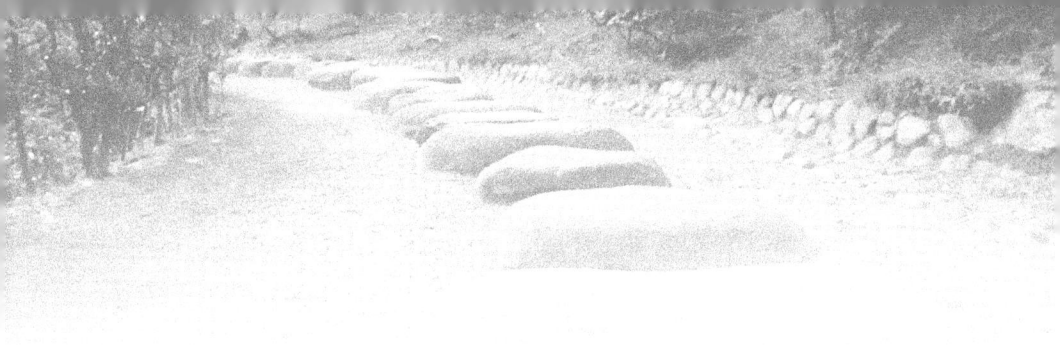

My Story

I believe that everyone has a unique story to tell. A story of struggles and victory. A tale of overcoming to become. My story is no different. While growing up, I had always struggled with my body image, which resulted in low self-esteem and a very introverted personality. I constantly compared myself with others and thought, "I'm not good enough" or "I'm not smart enough." Books were my best friends, and the library was my second home. I became a bookworm.

How many of you can relate to me? Mentally, I was on the road to disaster, going 100 miles an hour while faking smiles and happiness. My happiness depended on the scale, which is not an ideal way to live life.

Due to the lack of social support and proper knowledge, I had developed unhealthy eating habits in my teens and fallen into the trap of yo-yo diets. Also, I had seen my dad struggle with type 2 diabetes, which led me to my quest for extensive knowledge in health and wellness.

After completing my Master of Microbiology, along with my work, I continued my journey in search of optimal well-being by pursuing certification in the field of nutrition and healthy living from Cornell University. I walked away with some great information and knowledge after I earned the certificate, but, at the same time, I had some unanswered questions.

My main question was that if weight loss was as simple as calorie intake—calorie expenditure and creating a calorie deficit—why was it that everyone on the same diet and exercise routine, creating the same calorie deficit, did not lose the same amount of weight? At that point, I realized that weight loss depends not only on how much calorie deficit we create by our calorie expenditure but also on the quality of the calories. Calories from an excellent nutritious diet are not the same as calories from junk food.

This realization was an "aha" moment for me, but it was short-lived. I observed that two people on the same diet and exercise routine might have different weight-loss and wellness journeys. My point is that an individual's weight-loss or wellness journey is unique, and there is no cookie-cutter approach.

Also, several other factors, like hormones, inflammation, digestion, basal metabolic rate, an individual's environment, emotional well-being, socioeconomic condition, stress, quality of sleep, etc. These all play an essential role. Hence, I started my journey to learn Ayurveda, hoping that this ancient wisdom would answer my questions.

All the knowledge I've gained has helped me overcome my limitations, and today I have become confident in my skin. I have realized that God does not make any junk, and everyone has an inner genius. I know my self-worth and happiness do not depend on how I look or my material possessions but on my contributions to society. I love myself tremendously, and I know I am enough. Being healthy is a complete package that starts with a healthy soul, healthy mind, and healthy body.

By the grace of God, I have become victorious over unhealthy diet and exercise patterns. I have achieved a healthy body and radiant skin, a healthy mind, and high self-esteem. I am a passionate advocate for self-love, self-compassion, and healthy living through lifestyle changes, and I coach others to do the same. I know that lifestyle-related diseases can be healed by healthy habits and managing stress with excellent emotional health and a solid spiritual foundation.

I credit my growth to my critics, who always identified my value based on my looks and weight. Surprisingly enough, most of them were my near and dear ones. I bet everyone has critics in their social circle who make them feel that they are not enough.

Today, I challenge you to break those mental barriers created by your circle of influence and develop self-love. Surround yourself with people who love you and uplift you because of who you are, instead of how you look or what you have. Go ahead, find your cheerleader, and be a cheerleader for someone else. Your life will change for the better.

Have you heard of a term called kintsugi? It's the traditional Japanese art of using precious metal, like liquid gold, liquid silver, liquid platinum, or lacquer dusted with precious metal, to repair broken pottery, putting together the broken pieces, making it more beautiful and stronger. To me, kintsugi is the art of embracing our brokenness, or our wounds, and becoming stronger. I have been hammered several times by situations and people in my life, which shattered me into pieces. At the same time, I have learned the art of forgiveness, patience, unconditional love, and unconditional acceptance, which is my precious metal, and these have helped me heal my wounds.

Life has proven that no human is perfect and not to expect perfection from an imperfect human. The hammering of my life has shown me how much strength and wisdom I have. I am blessed by the glue that has held me together: my family, a few guides, and loyal friends, who have provided me with support and guidance. They taught me to forgive, be patient, and develop confidence in myself. I learned that I am enough, and I am capable. Now is the time for me to give back to others who are in a rough spot. Every day I strive to pay it forward and spread the hope that you can heal and believe that you, too, are enough.

Every day I see people trying hard to slow the effect of aging on their skin and hair and just trying to hold on to youth. But they have a firm grasp on an empty bag. Sometimes people go to the extent of trying crash diets to feel good about their bodies or use harmful chemicals on their faces to look younger and gain confidence. I am passionate about optimal well-being through making lifestyle changes by forming long-term sustainable habits and coaching others to do the same. During the darkest times in my life, the people in my support system stood by me to uplift and support me, hence now I strive to pay it forward and spread the hope so that you can heal and achieve your goals in all areas of your life. You are not alone on this journey. If you look around, there are people like me to support you.

Optimal well-being is the result of finding balance in all areas of life. Lifestyle changes are required to achieve optimal physical, emotional, spiritual, social, and financial well-being, and it all starts with showing some compassion and love toward oneself. People who can love themselves unconditionally and feel confident in their skin will love and accept others unconditionally.

This book gives you easy-to-follow and straightforward tips to start your journey toward optimal well-being and be comfortable in your skin. Just like it has for me, I hope this book will empower you to be victorious over any situation in your life. If you feel stuck at any point in your well-being journey, or you are looking for an accountability partner, email me at inquiries@krutithakore.com.

PART I

According to the World Health Organization (WHO), optimal well-being is the presence of life and health-giving practices like mindfulness, self-compassion, and self-love, proper habits that promote one to thrive in a life filled with energy.

Introduction

English is my third language, so I understand what it feels like for anyone who isn't fluent in the language. I have tried my best to keep the language in this book easy to understand so that anyone who isn't fluent in English can still read it and implement what they learn from the book. Also, I don't want to complicate the book's contents because it's hard to apply anything that confuses us. Confused people do not make decisions. Hence, I have followed the principle of keeping it simple.

The purpose of this book is to provide you with 12 easy-to-follow steps toward optimal well-being. It's a journey from *dis*ease to ease, from illness to wellness, and from hard to easy. So, fasten your seatbelts, as it's going to be an exciting ride.

Even though this book is for everyone, it is not meant to treat any serious illness, but was written to help you overcome minor fender benders in your life's journey, as I believe that prevention is better than cure. Today, we read statistics about the increase in metabolic syndrome disorders like increased body fat around the waist, increased blood sugar, increased blood pressure, and abnormal cholesterol levels that can lead to diabetes, hypertension, stroke, coronary artery disease, etc. We take pride in the scientific advancement that helps us and teaches us to live with these diseases. But we never think about preventing such lifestyle-related diseases from the get-go.

I have great respect for all the healthcare providers in the field of conventional medicine as they are in this noble field with a purpose to serve humanity and conventional medicine is equally important, as it helps in emergency and acute conditions, which can only be treated with medication or surgery. In the case of lifestyle-related illnesses, it helps curb the symptoms so that people can learn to manage them well. For example, once someone is on blood sugar medication, they will never get off it without changing their lifestyle. Also, conventional medicines can have a lot of side effects. This doesn't mean that you should stop medications given to you by your medical or healthcare practitioner, but when you follow the guidelines of this book along with taking your medicines, your body may respond to the medications in a better way, and you may have fewer side effects from these medicines. The steps in the book can also help you rebound faster after treatment of your acute condition is completed. You will notice that I have incorporated knowledge and practices from Ayurveda and holistic healing in this book. This is my effort to bring the best of both worlds to you.

We must understand that the quality of our lifestyle-related habits determines the quality of our life. It's the law of cause and effect or the law of action and reaction. One can also call it the law of karma or the law of sowing and reaping.

If you listen to the whispers of your body, you will never have to worry about the screams.

If you listen to the whispers of your body, you will never have to worry about the screams. The human body and mind together are highly intelligent, so if you become more mindful about how you live your life, you will improve the quality of your life.

Throughout this book, you will be exposed to the idea of being mindful, and you might wonder, what is mindfulness? Mindfulness means being consciously aware of your actions. It means not only are you aware of the choices you make, but you also become aware of the repercussions of the choices you make. You may spend more time thinking through your choices before you decide so that you make the right choices. You have a right to make choices in your life. Just make sure that you make the right choices.

Usually, people are mindful about significant decisions in their lives, like planning a vacation or a wedding, but are not as mindful about their day-to-day actions and thoughts. On a daily basis, people are creatures of habit, living mindlessly or on autopilot. They are not mindful of their negative thought patterns, the foods they eat, how much time they waste on social media, or how much money they waste on unnecessary stuff. These minor bad habits can come back to haunt you, as they determine the quality of your life.

Your date of birth and expiry date are always predetermined. The *quantity* of your life is not in your hands, but the *quality* of your life is in your hands because most illnesses are due to an unhealthy lifestyle. Hence, from today onward, take charge of your well-being because procrastination is the assassination of your dreams.

CHAPTER 1

What is Optimal Well-Being?

⫷⫷⫷

As per the dictionary, "optimal" means "most desirable or most favorable," and "well-being" means "the state of being healthy, happy, blissful, and prosperous." Hence, I feel that "optimal well-being" means "most desirable or most favorable state of being."

Optimal well-being is about the quality of your overall life. Not just about your physical health or emotional health. It can also mean a state of harmony, a state of equilibrium, or a state of balance.

Life becomes easy when we are in harmony with nature and the universe. We will achieve optimal well-being effortlessly. For some, optimal well-being might be just the absence of disease or illness, but, according to the World Health Organization (WHO), optimal well-being is the presence of life and health-giving practices like mindfulness, self-compassion, and self-love, proper habits that promote one to thrive in a life filled with energy. A person thrives when they tap into their unique strengths, skills, and talents to achieve their life's purpose by having a growth mindset and the ability to set and achieve goals by stretching and stepping out of their comfort zone.

Optimal well-being is multi-dimensional, and there is a strong correlation between optimal well-being and your lifestyle choices. Your ability to live life to the fullest depends on your optimal well-being, and your optimal well-being depends on how well you do in several dimensions and areas: physical, mental, emotional, spiritual, social, environmental, intellectual, occupational, and financial.

Optimal well-being is multi-dimensional, and there is a strong correlation between optimal well-being and your lifestyle choices.

There is a term in Sanskrit called "arogya," which means "overall well-being" or "well-being of mind, body, and spirit." All the dimensions mentioned above are critical and interconnected for the well-being of mind, body, and spirit. Our *arogya* is the foundation of all other pursuits in life. If someone is physically ill, they will not have the energy to pursue their goals, even if they have time, talent, intention, and resources. On the other hand, if someone is emotionally and mentally ill, their judgment and ability to make the right decisions, which would benefit not only them but their relationships and society, will be impaired, so they deviate from their true purpose.

When mind, body, and spirit are aligned, you can harness your true potential. In future chapters of this book, we shall see how all the dimensions of well-being affect each other; when one of these is impacted adversely, all others will be affected eventually, and a

When mind, body, and spirit are aligned, you can harness your true potential.

person will enter a state of discomfort or disease.

Now, let us look at what all these factors mean:

Physical Well-Being: Physical well-being means taking care of our physical body by a series of lifestyle choices so that we can avoid preventable illnesses. This is very crucial because, these days, people put premium gasoline in their automobiles but will put total junk in their bodies and mind. If your car breaks down, you can get another one. But what happens if your body breaks down?

Mental and Emotional Well-Being: According to the WHO: "There is no universally accepted 'definition' of mental well-being." This is probably because mental well-being may have different connotations for different individuals, groups, and cultures. For some, it may be the notion of happiness or contentment. For others, it may be the absence of disease. For some, it may be economic prosperity. It could be based on the goals sought to be achieved and the challenges placed on an individual or a culture. It also may mean the absence of negative determinants in the life of an individual or a community. Mental well-being includes cognitive, emotional, and behavioral responses at a personal level. In simple terms, mental and emotional well-being is the state of happiness, bliss, and peace. It determines how well we handle stress.

Spiritual Well-Being: There is no set definition of spiritual well-being either, but spiritual well-being means our ability to identify our purpose in life. Have a definiteness of purpose, and have a set of principles, values, and morals. Follow the path of righteousness by using intellect and consciousness to differentiate between good and evil. It also means having faith in a higher power, as it allows us to tune into our higher self as our anchor and gives us an inner sense of security. It provides us with the ability to stay hopeful during adverse circumstances. As Dr. Deepak Chopra says, "Each of us is here to discover our true selves; that essentially we are spiritual beings who have taken manifestation in physical form; that we're not human beings that have occasional spiritual experiences, that we're spiritual beings that have occasional human experiences."

I feel now is the perfect time to change our mindset and focus on improving our spiritual quotient (SQ). So far, we all have paid a lot of attention to IQ and EQ, but we have never focused on our SQ. The health of our soul depends on our SQ, and spiritual well-being is the most important dimension of our overall well-being. Spirituality teaches us humility and also helps to improve our self-confidence as it teaches us that no one is better than us, nor we are better than anyone else. We all are equal.

> *The health of our soul depends on our SQ, and spiritual well-being is the most important dimension of our overall well-being.*

Social Well-Being: Social well-being means our ability to create and maintain meaningful and positive relationships. Relationships play an essential role in our overall well-being, and our social well-being plays a vital role in the world's well-being. There is a Sanskrit phrase that explains this beautifully. "Vasudhaiva kutumbakam," which means "the world is one family." Another way to put this proverb is to say, "It takes a village to raise a child."

Our social responsibility is to create a safe society where our future generations can flourish and today's children feel safe so they can grow up to become responsible citizens of tomorrow. Our social well-being depends on our emotional and mental well-being because only an emotionally stable and happy person can give back to society and spread cheer and love.

Environmental Well-Being: Social well-being and environmental well-being go hand in hand. We all know the impact of our lifestyle on the environment of this planet. The scientific facts validate the effects of greenhouse gas emissions on global warming. Air, water, and soil pollution are man-made, and these impact our health drastically. Hence, as responsible human beings, we must do whatever it takes to reduce environmental pollution. You can contribute by recycling plastics and other recyclable materials, cutting down water and electricity usage, going solar, checking your car emissions, switching to an electric car instead of using gas guzzlers, using energy-efficient products, and green cleaning products in your house. After all, Mother Earth is our home, and we must keep it safe because our well-being and the well-being of future generations depend on environmental well-being.

Intellectual Well-Being: Intellectual well-being means our ability to pursue knowledge and skills. It also means our ability to discern between right and wrong, between good and evil, and between morality and immorality. There is a saying in India: "जैसी मति वैसी गति (jaisi mati taisi gati)," which means "The quality of your life depends on how you use your intellect."

Occupational and Financial Well-Being: Occupational well-being means one's ability to acquire the skills and talent that will help them create financial well-being and provide intellectual stimulation and fulfillment. In an ideal world, career growth and fulfillment depend on your capabilities, critical thinking, creativity, and ability to embrace new challenges, but there is a caveat. Finding passion in your job or occupation is not easy in today's competitive world, especially when you're overworked and underappreciated.

> *There is a saying in India: "जैसी मति वैसी गति (jaisi mati taisi gati)," which means "The quality of your life depends on how you use your intellect."*

Occupational well-being is compromised, as people live under constant pressure to outsmart their competition or fear losing their job. In short, ensure that your job or career does not become your identity because, God forbid, if you lose your job, you will feel lost and depressed, as if you have lost your identity and purpose in life. This is one more reason why there are so many people whose health deteriorates and age quickly after retirement. You are more than just your career since it is only one part of your overall life. You have hobbies, goals, friends, and family, all of which are a welcomed addition to your identity, over and above your career. Cultivate all aspects of your life in equal balance to ensure that you are a well-rounded individual. You are not defined by your job or by your material possessions. Your identity is defined by who you are as a human being and the value you offer to the world.

Have you heard of a Japanese concept called "Ikigai"? It is a field of unlimited potential, where; what you love meets, what you are good at, meets what you can be paid for, meets what the world needs. Ikigai is only complete if the goal implies service to the community. In other words, it can be explained as "our purpose" or "our dharma." In short, when there is alignment between our strengths, values, what the world needs, our passion, and our vision, our work does not feel like work. Work becomes fun, and we never feel the need to take a vacation from our work. This is when occupational well-being is achieved.

Work becomes fun, and we never feel the need to take a vacation from our work. This is when occupational well-being is achieved.

Occupational well-being and financial well-being are interconnected. Your occupation is one of the means to provide you with economic well-being, but it is not the only means. As per consumerfinance.gov, financial well-being means having financial security and freedom of choice in the present and the future.

References:

- *Prendergast, K. B., Schofield, G. M., & Mackay, L. M. (2016). Associations between lifestyle behaviors and optimal wellbeing in a diverse sample of New Zealand adults. BMC public health, 16, 62. https://www.ncbi.nlm.nih.gov/pmc/articles/PMC4722793/*
- *Bart, R., Ishak, W. W., Ganjian, S., Jaffer, K. Y., Abdelmesseh, M., Hanna, S., Gohar, Y., Azar, G., Vanle, B., Dang, J., & Danovitch, I. (2018). The Assessment and Measurement of Wellness in the Clinical Medical Setting: A Systematic Review. Innovations in clinical neuroscience, 15(9-10), 14–23. https://www.ncbi.nlm.nih.gov/pmc/articles/PMC6292717/*

CHAPTER 2

Why Strive for
Optimal Well-Being?

In his book *Think and Grow Rich*, Napoleon Hill mentioned that nothing could stop a human being who has definiteness of purpose from achieving their goals. A human being is bound to achieve all their goals when definiteness of purpose is backed by the definiteness of plans, burning desire, determination, willpower, self-discipline, mastermind alliance, and consistent and persistent efforts. Hence, it is crucial to identify why you want to achieve optimal well-being before going into the "how" of doing so.

My mentor always said, "Man without a dream shall perish." Anything worthwhile takes time and consistent and persistent effort. As they say, "Rome was not built in a day; it was built every day." Your "why" or dreams will give you the willpower to be consistent and persistent in your pursuit of optimal well-being.

Everyone is unique, and so is their "why." For some, it would be to improve the quality of their life or to age healthily. There might be some people who want to get off diabetes medicine, while someone else might want to enjoy an active life with their kids and grandkids. You might be sick and tired of the stress and cannot take the lack of work-life balance. You must figure out how you want to live the rest of your life. Write down those goals before you read the rest of this book and identify your "why" because where there is a will, there is a way.

Your "why" or dreams will give you the willpower to be consistent and persistent in your pursuit of optimal well-being.

The quality of your life depends on how well you are doing in all the dimensions of well-being mentioned in the previous chapter. Your ability to manage daily stress, your mental attitude, how you respond to any situation, your contribution to relationships and society, and your ability to live life to the fullest depend on your optimal well-being.

It is essential to strive to achieve wellness in all the areas mentioned above, as they are all interconnected. When you are building a luxurious, multimillion-dollar mansion, you make sure that all the walls of its foundation are solid and well-built so that they can support the massive structure. Your life is more valuable than a luxurious, multimillion-dollar mansion. All the dimensions of well-being mentioned in the previous chapter are the walls of the foundation of the mansion of your life. If one wall is weak, or if it falls apart, all other walls will have to bear the load, and, eventually, they will also become weak, and the mansion of your life will crumble.

For example, if you have a lifestyle-related illness, it will affect your sleep and productivity during the day. When someone doesn't get a good night's sleep, they feel tired and lethargic the next day. This increases stress, and they may become agitated. They may tend to make a mountain out of a molehill and snap at others. Also, they may make poor food choices or eat out because they don't have the energy to fix a balanced meal, nor do they have the energy to exercise. All these factors will have more impact on their physical health, as well as social and emotional health. Very soon, productivity at work is reduced, and finances are now impacted. It becomes a vicious cycle, and so it is essential to have a balanced approach and focus on achieving well-being in all dimensions.

I recommend that you journal 12 reasons why you want to achieve optimal well-being.

CHAPTER 3

What is Ayurveda?

Charaka Sutra Sthana, Chapter 1, verse 41

हिताहितं सुखं दुःखमायुस्तस्य हिताहितम्‌|
मानं च तच्च यत्रोक्तमायुर्वेदः स उच्यते||४१||

Hitahitam sukham dukhamayustasya hitahitam
Maanam cha tacha yatrokatmayurvedah sa uchyate

Ayurveda is the science of life. Ayurveda gives remedies for…
Hitayu – an advantageous life
Ahita ayu – a disadvantageous life
Sukhayu – a happy state of health and mind
Ahitayu – an unhappy state of health and mind.

Ayurveda also explains what is good and bad for life and how to improve the quality of life. It is the world's most sophisticated mind-body health system, a 5000-year-old ancient healing system based on Vedic principles. Ayurveda, the original lifestyle and personalized medicine, is the best gift from

Ayurveda, the original lifestyle and personalized medicine, is the best gift from India to the world.

India to the world. Of the four main Vedas— Rig Veda, Sam Veda, Yajur Veda, and Atharv Veda—Ayurveda is upveda (part of) of Atharv Veda. It originated in ancient India, and the knowledge was passed down verbally by the sages from generations before it was documented in Sanskrit in the form of mantras and sutras (verses).

Sages of India developed the concept of interrelation between mind, body, spirit, and environment thousands of years before modern medicine acknowledged the connection. The meaning of Ayurveda is "wisdom of life" and is derived from "ayus" (life) and "Veda" (wisdom/knowledge/science).

In addition to Atharv Veda, there are two other reference texts:

- **Charaka Samhita**, which covers Ayurvedic internal medicine, physiology, disease, herbal formulations, detoxification, panchakarma, and rejuvenation therapies.
- **Sushruta Samhita**, which covers details about surgery, including surgical procedures, cleaning and disinfecting surgical instruments, and anesthesia.

Sages of India developed the concept of interrelation between mind, body, spirit, and environment thousands of years before modern medicine acknowledged the connection.

Historians and scholars estimate that these texts were written somewhere between 700 and 100 BCE.

Ayurveda is a holistic approach to healing. It focuses on prevention and encourages the maintenance of optimal health through creating harmony in life between mind, body, soul, and environment. It is a consciousness-based approach, and its purpose is to empower us to reach an optimal state of well-being. It's about experiencing the changes in our mind, body, soul, and environment by making positive choices about food, personal relationships, thoughts, experiences, sleep, work, social interactions, and daily routine. It focuses on living in harmony with other human beings, as well as with nature.

The knowledge of this ancient wisdom teaches us to create a balance between mind, body, and consciousness, according to one's unique mind-body constitution (dosha), through lifestyle changes and daily routines; to attain a state of optimal well-being. This book on optimal wellness would be incomplete without sharing this ancient Vedic wisdom because it explains the fundamental truth of the universe: that our mind, body, soul, and environment are interconnected and, also, we all are connected with each other, as well as with the Supreme Power, which some call God, while others call "higher intelligence."

To explain this concept in simple terms, we can use the analogy of the ocean and the waves. When a wave comes to the shore, it is individual but still has all the properties of the ocean. The same is true for all waves, no matter the size of the wave. They all have the same fundamental property of the ocean, and once the wave returns to the ocean, it becomes one with the ocean. Thus, every wave has its individuality and uniqueness; at the same time, all waves are interconnected with each other, as well as with the ocean. The same is true for all creatures in the universe.

Ayurveda is the original form of lifestyle or integrative medicine. Several studies in integrative medicine have shown that approximately 90 percent of chronic illnesses can be prevented and even reversed by making the right lifestyle choices daily. Ayurveda and other holistic approaches have tools and guidance to help you achieve this goal. At the same time, we must not undermine the importance of modern medical science, as Ayurveda believes that we should use whatever is available to support healing.

In integrative medicine practices like Ayurveda, while treating anyone, the focus is not just on the symptom but also on the root cause of the disease. The body, mind, soul, and environment are considered one unit, and to be genuinely healthy, optimal health in all the areas of life is required. Our physical body cannot be healthy if we do not focus on the health of mind, spirit, and the environment, as all these aspects are interconnected. We can experience the state of optimal well-being only by addressing the needs of mind, body, soul, and environment.

References:

- *Sharma, H. (2016). Ayurveda: Science of life, genetics, and epigenetics. Ayu. https://www.ncbi.nlm.nih.gov/pubmed/29200745.*
- *Chatterjee, B., & Pancholi, J. (2011, April). Prakriti-based medicine: A step toward personalized medicine. Ayu. https://www.ncbi.nlm.nih.gov/pubmed/22408293.*
- *Thakar V. J. (2010). Historical development of basic concepts of Ayurveda from Veda up to Samhita. Ayu, 31(4), 400–402. https://doi.org/10.4103/0974-8520.82024*
- *Chauhan, A., Semwal, D. K., Mishra, S. P., & Semwal, R. B. (2015). Ayurvedic research and methodology: Present status and future strategies. Ayu. https://www.ncbi.nlm.nih.gov/pmc/articles/PMC5041382/*

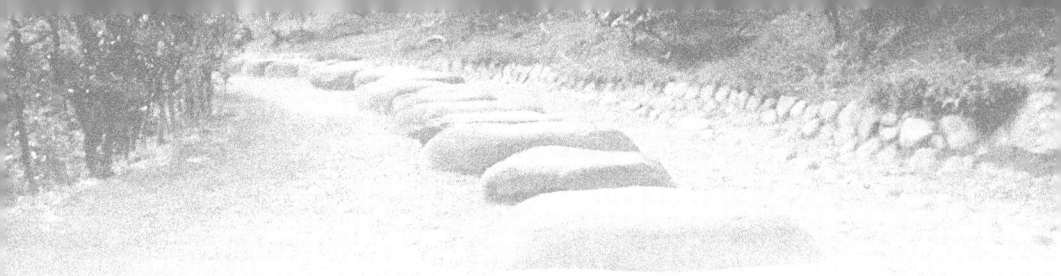

CHAPTER 4

East Meets West

❦

In this chapter, we shall understand the fundamental difference between integrative holistic medicine practices, like Ayurveda and conventional medicine. In addition to Ayurveda, other integrative medicine practices are homeopathy, acupuncture, acupressure, naturopathy, oriental medicine, chiropractic treatment, Yunani medicine, etc.

Ayurveda is an ancient science and has a rich history. The basic principles of Ayurveda are applicable and valid even today. People use many Ayurvedic remedies as home remedies or "grandma's remedies." While conventional medicine is a symptom-centric cure, Ayurvedic medicine is preventative and person-centric. Ayurveda and conventional medicine both are important as they have their own purpose in healing. Ayurveda is a strong advocate for a healthy lifestyle and disease prevention, as the holistic principles of Ayurveda focus on early diagnosis, personalized treatment, prevention, and living in harmony with nature. I had experienced many benefits from Ayurvedic practices, like panchakarma and Ayurvedic nutrition, and detoxification for my allergy problems when conventional medical science did not offer any help. After all the allergy medicines and immunotherapy failed, my doctor recommended surgery for nasal polyps and a deviated septum, so I tried Ayurvedic practices as a last resort to prevent surgery.

While conventional medical science treats by focusing on symptoms and disease, lifestyle medicines, like Ayurveda, focus on healing by treating the root cause of the disease. For example, if a patient suffers from hyperacidity, an allopathic physician might prescribe a standard course of antacids and, perhaps, change the diet. On the other hand, an Ayurvedic doctor would seek to understand the root cause and dosha imbalances that are causing the problem. An Ayurvedic doctor would consider the patient's mind, body, spirit, and environment. They would also consider the patient's lifestyle, activities, diet, recent stressful events, beliefs, and mind-body constitution and recommend a treatment plan to address the root cause of the acidity by taking all these factors into account. So, for an allopathic physician, hyperacidity is the *problem*. For an Ayurvedic physician, hyperacidity is the *symptom* of other imbalances in the body.

> *While conventional medicine is a symptom-centric cure, Ayurvedic medicine is preventative and person-centric.*

I want to add here that Ayurveda accepts the use of antacids to give relief to the patient but, at the same time, looks to heal the root cause of the hyperacidity in the first place. Hence, I feel Ayurveda starts where conventional medicine ends.

As modern medicine has failed us in several ways, some doctors turn to functional medicine or integrative medicine for answers. Ayurveda is an essential component of integrative, or functional, medicine where the focus is on the whole person, including mind, body, spirit, and environment, instead of just the disease. In this patient-centric approach, each patient care plan is distinct and unique. There is no one-size-fits-all approach. The belief here is that poor lifestyle habits are the root cause of all chronic diseases. Hence, the practitioner partners with the patient by becoming a coach and a mentor to empower and promote healthy lifestyle changes. The purpose of this book is to bring the best of ayurvedic practices and conventional medicine.

As a perfect health Ayurvedic lifestyle instructor and NBC-HWC, Board-certified health coach, National Board of Health, and wellness coaching, my focus is on empowering and inspiring my clients to change their lifestyle so that they can achieve optimal well-being. Along with the certification from The Chopra Center in Perfect Health Ayurvedic Lifestyle, my education in microbiology and certifications in integrative health and well-being from YogamedCo, as well as in nutrition and healthy living from Cornell, has empowered me to bring the best of both the worlds to the table for my clients.

References:

- *Morandi, A., Tosto, C., Sartori, G., & Roberti di Sarsina, P. (2011). Advent of a Link between Ayurveda and Modern Health Science: The Proceedings of the First International Congress on Ayurveda, "Ayurveda: The Meaning of Life-Awareness, Environment, and Health" March 21-22, 2009, Milan, Italy. Evidence-based complementary and alternative medicine: eCAM. https://www.ncbi.nlm.nih.gov/pubmed/20981327.*
- *Patwardhan, B. (2014, November 1). Bridging Ayurveda with evidence-based scientific approaches in medicine. The EPMA journal. https://www.ncbi.nlm.nih.gov/pmc/articles/PMC4230501/.*

CHAPTER 5

Endocrine System and Our Hormones

The miraculous human body is more sophisticated and complicated than most advanced chemical plants in the world. The endocrine system is the network of glands and organs in our body that uses chemical messengers—called hormones—to communicate and conduct bodily functions. It produces several hormones, steroids, and enzymes to perform physiological and psychological functions. These hormones are released into and transported via our circulatory system to target and govern the functions of our organs. It controls functions like growth, metabolism, reproduction, mood, hunger, sleep, respiration, movement, sexual development, etc.

The miraculous human body is more sophisticated and complicated than most advanced chemical plants in the world.

Enzymes act as a catalyst for a reaction, while hormones act as a messenger to send messages to trigger bodily functions. Steroids are hormones or chemicals similar to hormones but may have different functions.

We will not discuss all the hormones, enzymes, and steroids produced by the human body, but we will discuss the role of a few of them and how they affect our well-being. This doesn't mean that the rest of them don't matter. Maintaining an optimal balance of all the chemicals in our body is crucial for our well-being because our hormones are responsible for essentially every function in our bodies.

When your hormones are balanced and working in sync, your body is in a state of homeostasis,[1] which is a good thing. At the same time, when they're imbalanced, you may start experiencing health challenges. Also, as you read further in this book, you will understand how these 12 steps to optimal well-being will help you balance your hormones. But, before that, let us learn about the functions of our endocrine system and some of these hormones.

The glands of the endocrine system that produce hormones are:

Hypothalamus: Located in the base of the brain above the pituitary gland. Produces multiple hormones to control the pituitary gland. Responsible for body temperature, hunger, thirst, mood, sleep-wake cycles, sex drive.

Pituitary: Located below the hypothalamus is the "boss" or "master," as it controls the function of other glands and affects the function of every part of your body. The hormones it produces regulate growth, reproduction, sex drive, milk production in new mothers, etc.

---

1   Definition of homeostasis: A property of cells, tissues, and organisms that allows the maintenance and regulation of the stability and constancy needed to function correctly. Homeostasis is a healthy state maintained by the constant adjustment of biochemical and physiological pathways.

Pineal: Located deep in the brain, the pineal gland is responsible for sleep-wake cycles. It receives dark and light signals from the environment and secretes melatonin, which slows down bodily functions and prepares you for a good night's sleep. It also affects your ability to respond to stress and controls your body's biorhythms. It is believed to be associated with Ajna Chakra or your third eye in the spiritual world. Currently, much research is being done on the pineal gland to see its impact on mood, psychological disorders, and cardiovascular health.

Thyroid: This butterfly-shaped gland, located in the front part of your neck, releases hormones that control metabolism, growth, and development.

Parathyroid: Produces hormones that regulate calcium levels in your blood and bones, as precise calcium levels are vital for the smooth functioning of our bodies.

Thymus: Located below the breastbone, this is an essential organ for developing a healthy immune system. It produces T cells, which play a vital role in developing and maintaining the immune system. They also help us prevent cancer by destroying cancerous cells. It is only active until you hit puberty and functions as an endocrine gland and lymphatic gland.

Adrenal: Located right above the kidneys, adrenal glands are a group of two glands: the adrenal cortex and adrenal medulla. They produce cortisol (which regulates metabolism, i.e., how our body converts fats, proteins, and carbohydrates into energy; it also regulates our body's response to stress), aldosterone (helps to control blood pressure), and adrenaline (which helps the body react to stress by preparing for "fight or flight").

Pancreas: Located behind your stomach, the pancreas plays a vital role in digestion by making enzymes called lipase, protease, and amylase, which are responsible for the breakdown of fats, proteins, and carbohydrates. They also manufacture hormones and help regulate blood sugar levels, appetite, stimulate the production of gastric acids, and control the emptying of the stomach.

Ovaries and testes: These reproductive organs are also considered endocrine glands. They are responsible for producing ovum (ovaries) and sperm (testes), as well as sex hormones. They play a vital role in reproduction.

Here are a few hormones, enzymes, and their functions:

Mucoproteins: These have various functions, ranging from determination of immune properties, blood group affiliation, elasticity, and permeability of membranes. Also, a critical function of mucoproteins is to coat your stomach before you eat to protect your stomach lining from digestive acid or stomach acid. Your parasympathetic nervous system is responsible for the activation of these mucoproteins. Hence, it is essential not to consume food under stress or when your sympathetic nervous system is active. We shall discuss the roles of the sympathetic nervous system, parasympathetic nervous system, and the importance of mindful eating in later chapters.

Gastrin: The parasympathetic nervous system activates G-cells in the stomach and upper small intestine lining to produce a powerful hormone called gastrin. Gastrin's role is to stimulate the cells of your stomach to produce stomach acid. It also helps the pancreas produce enzymes for digestion and stimulates the liver to produce bile. Thus, it plays a vital role in the digestion of food.

Amylin: A peptide hormone that is secreted by the pancreas, along with insulin. It is a neuroendocrine hormone that plays a vital role in glucose regulation by inhibiting glucagon secretion, delaying gastric emptying, and sending satiety signals to the brain.

Cholecystokinin (CCK): CCK aids in the release of digestive enzymes and hormones from the pancreas, which breaks down carbohydrates, fats, and proteins. It also plays a vital role in the secretion of bile.

Secretin: Secretin regulates secretions of the stomach, pancreas, and liver and plays a vital role in neutralizing acid contents flowing from the stomach because the rest of the gastrointestinal tract cannot handle this acid.

Insulin: Insulin is a hormone released by the pancreas that regulates blood sugar levels. Insulin, along with amylin, helps to reduce post-meal glucose levels by stimulating your muscle tissue and fat cells to absorb glucose from the bloodstream, where it is converted to fat and stored for future purposes. Thus, these two hormones play a vital role in maintaining blood sugar levels and reducing the amount of glucose dumped into your liver. At the same time, remember that excess sugar will be converted to fat and stored for future use. When insulin is around, glucose is stored as fat in the fat cells, but, at the same time, it stops the release of fat from fat cells in the form of energy. In short, the more glucose in the bloodstream, the more insulin is released, and more insulin more fat is stored in the fat cells. This results in highly sensitive insulin receptors. When insulin receptors are sensitive, they pull more glucose into fat cells to be stored as fat. This will result in an increased size of fat cells. Though we are not going into minute detail about glucose metabolism, it is essential to understand that a sugar- and carb-rich diet can lead to obesity, diabetes, and fatty liver syndrome. Hence, it is crucial to develop a habit of mindful eating. We shall review the topic of mindful eating in later chapters of the book.

Also, it is imperative to keep moving because the mechanism of glucose absorption in your muscle tissue is different from that in your fat cells. The absorption of glucose by your muscles is activated by movement. So, the more active you are, the more glucose your muscle tissues pick up to convert into energy to support your active lifestyle. We will review the benefits of mindful movement in later chapters of this book.

Ideal fasting blood glucose levels should be below 100 mg/dL. Fasting blood sugar levels between 100 mg/dL and 125 mg/dL are considered prediabetic, while people with fasting blood sugar levels higher than 125 mg/dL are considered diabetic.

If diabetes is a disease and is terrible, then why, you might wonder, does your body produce glucose or need glucose? The body converts the meals we eat into their simplest form, glucose, to produce energy, which is broken down into "ATP" through a series of biochemical reactions. ATP is the energy currency required by our body to perform biological activities. Glucose is required because it can easily be converted into ATP, but, at the same time, excess glucose is *not* good because when there is too much glucose in the bloodstream, it can penetrate the neural tissues in your body. All the carbohydrates are converted into glucose, while approximately 50 percent to 60 percent of protein is converted into glucose. Very little fat is converted to glucose.

Ideal fasting blood glucose levels should be below 100 mg/dL. Fasting blood sugar levels between 100 mg/dL and 125 mg/dL are considered prediabetic, while people with fasting blood sugar levels higher than 125 mg/dL are considered diabetic.

Neural tissues are present in various parts of your body. These tissues don't have mechanisms to convert excess glucose into fat for storage. Hence, the glucose here is converted into other forms of sugar, like fructose and sorbitol. Once they are formed, they cannot leave the neural tissues, and they cause dysfunction in these tissues through conditions like double vision, foot ulcers, excess buildup of fat and cholesterol in arteries, etc.

Glucagon: Along with insulin, glucagon helps maintain blood sugar levels. If blood sugar levels drop below 60–50 mg/dL, glucagon is activated, which will work on the glycogen stored in the liver and convert it into glucose to regulate blood sugar levels.

Leptin: There is much research being done on leptin and ghrelin. Leptin and ghrelin play a crucial role in obesity and fat storage. Leptin is produced by your fat cells, and its function is to tell the hypothalamus in your brain that you have enough fat stored in the body; hence you do not need to eat. It regulates how many calories you eat and store along with regulating energy intake and expenditure. High levels of leptin tell your brain that you have enough fat stored, and it does not need to store more fat. Low leptin levels tell your brain that you need to eat and store fat. In short, leptin is your satiety hormone.

Now, looking at this math, you might think that people who are obese would have high levels of leptin because it is produced by fat cells. The more fat, the more leptin. So, it should be easy for them to eat less and spend more, but sometimes this is not true. Even when there are high leptin levels in the body, the brain does not get signals to eat fewer calories and spend more calories because of leptin resistance.[2] Also, when someone consumes empty calories by eating junk food, the body does not get the nutrition it needs to function properly, so it craves more food.

Sugar, processed food, junk food, stress, and unhealthy lifestyle habits cause leptin resistance. Also, fad diets promote leptin

---

2   Leptin resistance is a condition where your brain does not get the signal to recognize the presence of leptin, so it does not feel full. Leptin resistance can cause people to take in more calories and spend fewer.

supplements, but research has yet to prove their effectiveness. At the same time, some supplements, like fiber, conjugated linoleic acid, alpha-lipoic acid, green tea extract (like ECGC), and fish oil may help you reduce leptin resistance when used in addition to lifestyle changes, like getting a good night's sleep (as per circadian rhythms discussed in later chapters); consuming a healthy diet (filled with lean protein, fiber, whole grains, leafy greens); and incorporating exercise into your daily routine. We shall discuss this in more detail in our chapters on the pillars of well-being.

Sugar, processed food, junk food, stress, and unhealthy lifestyle habits cause leptin resistance.

Leptin is one more reason why diet plans don't always work for the long term. Diet plans may help you lose fat, but, at the same time, this results in a reduction of leptin, which results in increased appetite and low motivation to exercise. As a result, your body starts storing fat because your brain thinks you are starving, resulting in changed behavior, like reduced basal metabolic rate, low motivation, and increased hunger.

Ghrelin: This is produced in your gut and is also called the hunger hormone. It travels to the brain through the bloodstream, and it signals to your brain to increase your appetite and consume food. This is one more reason long-term diet plans don't work. Research shows that most dieters regain weight and fat because the levels of ghrelin increase in their bodies when they are on a diet, and it becomes hard for them to continue their diet journey, resulting in yo-yo diet patterns. Also, consumption of sugar, processed food, fast food, junk food, stress, and unhealthy lifestyle habits will increase ghrelin levels in your body. You can reduce ghrelin levels by incorporating whole grains, fiber, protein, and healthy fat in your diet, along with working toward reducing stress and increasing muscle mass by exercising.

Thyroid hormones (T3 & T4): The thyroid gland uses iodine from your food and produces thyroid hormones T3 and T4, which play a significant role in regulating the metabolism of every cell in your body. They also regulate the rate at which your body burns calories in addition to regulating body temperature and heart rate, and several other metabolic functions.

Estrogen, progesterone, and testosterone are male and female sex hormones. They play a significant role in sexual and reproductive development.

HGH: Human growth hormones (HGH) are responsible for growth, boosting muscle and bone growth, body composition, regulation of body fluids, regulation of fat metabolism, increasing exercise performance, and improving recovery from injuries. Optimal HGH levels are essential in weight loss, enhancing exercise performance, and recovering quickly from injuries. Research says that living a healthy lifestyle, like eliminating sugar and junk food from your diet, managing stress well, getting enough sleep, intermittent fasting, not eating before bedtime, and exercising at high intensity, can improve your HGH levels.

> *Optimal HGH levels are essential in weight loss, enhancing exercise performance, and recovering quickly from injuries.*

Melatonin: Melatonin is produced by our brain in response to darkness. It is called the "hormone of darkness." It impacts your sleep-wake cycle and helps you improve the quality of your sleep.

Stress hormones (adrenaline, cortisol, norepinephrine): As per the National Institute of Health, "'Stress' may be defined as any situation which tends to disturb the equilibrium between a living organism and its environment." In the event of stress, our sympathetic nervous system is active, and our body releases stress hormones in response to stress. It is your body's alarm system, in response to any threat, to generate a "flight or fight response." The fight or flight response was created to protect us, but when we experience constant stress, the stress hormones cause inflammation, increased blood pressure and blood sugar levels, alter the immune response, and suppress digestive functions, the reproductive system, and growth functions.

As per the National Institute of Health, "'Stress' may be defined as any situation which tends to disturb the equilibrium between a living organism and its environment."

Happy hormones (serotonin, dopamine, oxytocin, and endorphins): These promote positive feelings like joy, peace, happiness, and love. They also help reduce chronic inflammation. The pillars of well-being discussed later in this book will help you increase happy hormones and reduce stress hormones.

References:

- *Billman GE. Homeostasis: The Underappreciated and Far Too Often Ignored Central Organizing Principle of Physiology. Front Physiol. 2020 Mar 10;11:200. doi: 10.3389/fphys.2020.00200. PMID: 32210840; PMCID: PMC7076167. https://pubmed.ncbi.nlm.nih.gov/32210840/*

- *Campbell M, Jialal I. Physiology, Endocrine Hormones. [Updated 2021 Oct 1]. In: StatPearls [Internet]. Treasure Island (FL): StatPearls Publishing; 2021 Jan-. Available from: https://www.ncbi.nlm.nih.gov/books/NBK538498/*

- *Hiller-Sturmhöfel S, Bartke A. The endocrine system: an overview. Alcohol Health Res World. 1998;22(3):153-64. PMID: 15706790; PMCID: PMC6761896. Available from: https://www.ncbi.nlm.nih.gov/pmc/articles/PMC6761896/*

- *Hannibal, K. E., & Bishop, M. D. (2014). Chronic stress, cortisol dysfunction, and pain: a psychoneuroendocrine rationale for stress management in pain rehabilitation. Physical therapy, 94(12), 1816–1825. https://www.ncbi.nlm.nih.gov/pmc/articles/PMC4263906/*

- *Liu, Y. Z., Wang, Y. X., & Jiang, C. L. (2017). Inflammation: The Common Pathway of Stress-Related Diseases. Frontiers in human neuroscience, 11, 316. https://www.ncbi.nlm.nih.gov/pmc/articles/PMC5476783/*

CHAPTER 6

Vagus Nerve, Sympathetic & Parasympathetic Nervous Systems

※≪≪

As we saw in our earlier chapter, the digestion of the food we intake and several other biological functions is supported well when your parasympathetic nervous system is activated. Your sympathetic nervous system is responsible for the flight or fight response and is activated under any stress or threat. In contrast, the parasympathetic nervous system, which is responsible for rest and repair, is activated when you are calm and at peace.

The sympathetic nervous system and the parasympathetic nervous system represent two of the three branches of the autonomic nervous system. The vagus nerve is the main contributor to the parasympathetic nervous system and is the longest of the 10 cranial nerves in the human body. This nerve originates in the brain and extends to the digestive tract through the neck and thorax. Its job is to carry signals from the brain to your digestive system, as well as other organs, and vice versa. It is responsible for the mind-body connection. Your vagus nerve regulates internal organ functions, such as heart rate, respiratory rate, digestion, dilation of blood vessels, stimulation of salivary glands, and reflex actions, such as coughing, sneezing, swallowing, and vomiting.

When the vagus nerve is stimulated, your brain sends signals of calm, relaxation, repair, and rejuvenation to your body. Hence, it is the most crucial nerve for creating long-term well-being, resilience, and rejuvenation. Several studies have shown that vagus nerve stimulation has promising results in treating post-traumatic stress disorder. It lowers the heart rate, reduces blood pressure, boosts immunity, improves digestion, heals several lifestyle-related illnesses, reduces depression and anxiety, and cures irritable bowel syndrome. Vagus nerve stimulation can reduce chronic inflammation and initiate your body's relaxation response. Thus, the vagus nerve is your key to ultimate well-being.

When the vagus nerve is stimulated, your brain sends signals of calm, relaxation, repair, and rejuvenation to your body.

Our ancestors were hunter-gatherers, and the sympathetic nervous system played an essential role in protecting them from the dangers of the wild. These days, our fast life, unhealthy eating habits, corporate competition, and the habit of living life on the edge unnecessarily put the sympathetic nervous system in overdrive mode. Symptoms of an overactive sympathetic nervous system are anxiety, insomnia, nervousness, breathlessness, panic, rapid heart palpitations, jittery feelings, inability to sit still or stay calm, and high cholesterol, to name a few.

Thus, an overactive sympathetic nervous system leads to chronic inflammation.

Research has shown that chronic inflammation is responsible for lifestyle-related diseases like high blood pressure, coronary artery disease, heart failures, stroke, diabetes, autoimmune diseases, compromised immunity, irritable bowel syndrome, and many more. We need to understand the difference between acute inflammation and chronic inflammation. Acute inflammation occurs only for a short period. Its purpose is to heal a part of the body, and it subsides once the job is done. It is suitable for our bodies. But, when our body is in a constant state of stress at a cellular level, we experience *chronic* inflammation, which is deleterious for our health.

Hence, you must learn to activate the parasympathetic nervous system to restore the body to a calm and relaxed state. When the sympathetic nervous system is activated, your heartbeats and respiration levels will increase; blood rushes to large muscle groups, like arms and legs; and digestion slows down. When the parasympathetic nervous system is activated, it slows down respiration and heartbeats while improving digestion, relaxation, and repair. When the parasympathetic nervous system is activated, it causes dilation of blood vessels and bronchioles in the lungs and stimulates salivary glands. On the contrary, the sympathetic nervous system constricts blood vessels and bronchioles and increases the heart rate.

My 12 steps to optimal well-being will give you a complete guideline to keep your sympathetic nervous system under check by learning healthy stress management techniques and help you activate your parasympathetic nervous system and vagus nerve to promote repair and restoration so that you can achieve optimal well-being.

References:

- Breit S., Kupferberg A., Rogler G., Hasler G. *Vagus Nerve as Modulator of the Brain-Gut Axis in Psychiatric and Inflammatory Disorders. Front Psychiatry. 2018 Mar 13;9:44. doi: 10.3389/fpsyt.2018.00044. PMID: 29593576; PMCID: PMC5859128. Available from: https://www.ncbi.nlm.nih.gov/pmc/articles/PMC5859128/*

- Howland R. H. (2014). *Vagus Nerve Stimulation. Current behavioral neuroscience reports, 1(2), 64–73. https://www.ncbi.nlm.nih.gov/pmc/articles/PMC4017164/*

- Kwan, H., Garzoni, L., Liu, H. L., Cao, M., Desrochers, A., Fecteau, G., Burns, P., & Frasch, M. G. (2016). *Vagus Nerve Stimulation for Treatment of Inflammation: Systematic Review of Animal Models and Clinical Studies. Bioelectronic medicine, 3, 1–6. https://www.ncbi.nlm.nih.gov/pmc/articles/PMC5063949/*

- Chopra, D. D., Kshirsagar, D. S., Simon, D. D., Patel, D. S., Porter, D. V., Saint, D. M., Gabriel, R., Stern, E., & Nadarajah, M. (2019, November). *The perfect health ayurvedic lifestyle online enrichment program. Session 1–15.*

- Johnson RL, Wilson CG. *A review of vagus nerve stimulation as a therapeutic intervention. J Inflamm Res. 2018 May 16;11:203–213. doi: 10.2147/JIR.S163248. PMID: 29844694; PMCID: PMC5961632. https://pubmed.ncbi.nlm.nih.gov/29844694/*

- Bonaz, B., Sinniger, V., & Pellissier, S. (2016). *Anti-inflammatory properties of the vagus nerve: potential therapeutic implications of vagus nerve stimulation. The Journal of Physiology, 594(20), 5781–5790. https://www.ncbi.nlm.nih.gov/pmc/articles/PMC5063949/*

- Waxenbaum JA, Reddy V, Varacallo M. *Anatomy, Autonomic Nervous System. [Updated 2021 Jul 29]. In: StatPearls [Internet]. Treasure Island (FL): StatPearls Publishing; 2022 Jan-. Available from: https://www.ncbi.nlm.nih.gov/books/NBK539845/*

CHAPTER 7

Macronutrients

‹‹‹‹

The two types of nutrients that our bodies use to perform biological functions are macronutrients and micronutrients. In this chapter, we will learn about macronutrients. Macronutrients are essential for proper body functioning, and the body requires large amounts of them. All macronutrients must be obtained through diet; the body cannot produce macronutrients on its own. Macronutrients are carbohydrates, proteins, and fats.

The Harvard's Healthy Eating Plate mentioned on the following page is the general guideline for macronutrient consumption. We will discuss more details in our chapter on nutrition and mindful eating.

Carbohydrates:

What are carbohydrates? Carbohydrates are the sugars, starches, and fibers found in fruits, grains, vegetables, and milk products. They are macronutrients, like proteins and fats, and are one of the three main ways our bodies obtain energy. They are called carbohydrates because the chemical composition of carbohydrates is made up of carbon, hydrogen, and oxygen molecules. 50 percent to 60 percent

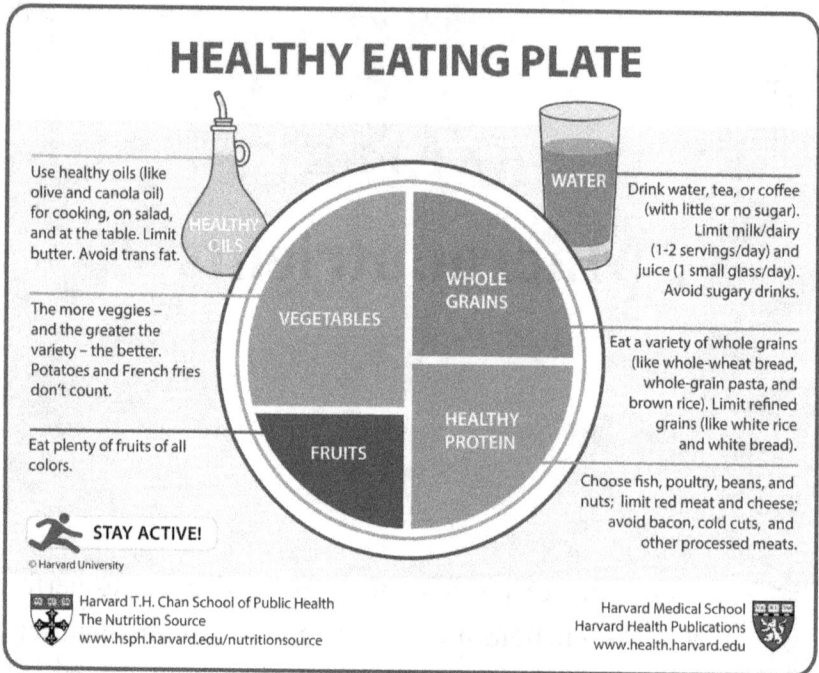

HEALTHY EATING PLATE

Use healthy oils (like olive and canola oil) for cooking, on salad, and at the table. Limit butter. Avoid trans fat.

HEALTHY OILS

WATER

Drink water, tea, or coffee (with little or no sugar). Limit milk/dairy (1-2 servings/day) and juice (1 small glass/day). Avoid sugary drinks.

VEGETABLES

WHOLE GRAINS

The more veggies – and the greater the variety – the better. Potatoes and French fries don't count.

Eat a variety of whole grains (like whole-wheat bread, whole-grain pasta, and brown rice). Limit refined grains (like white rice and white bread).

FRUITS

HEALTHY PROTEIN

Eat plenty of fruits of all colors.

Choose fish, poultry, beans, and nuts; limit red meat and cheese; avoid bacon, cold cuts, and other processed meats.

STAY ACTIVE!

© Harvard University

Harvard T.H. Chan School of Public Health
The Nutrition Source
www.hsph.harvard.edu/nutritionsource

Harvard Medical School
Harvard Health Publications
www.health.harvard.edu

"Copyright © 2011 Harvard University. For more information about The Healthy Eating Plate, please see The Nutrition Source, Department of Nutrition, Harvard T.H. Chan School of Public Health, http://www.thenutritionsource.org and Harvard Health Publications, health.harvard.edu."

of the calories we eat should come from carbohydrates. We consume carbohydrates as they are an excellent source of energy. ATP[1] (adenosine triphosphate), is the energy-carrying molecule; the only form of energy our bodies can use. Hence, whatever we eat must be converted to ATP through various biological mechanisms.

Carbohydrates come in three different forms. Monosaccharides

---

1   ATP (adenosine triphosphate) is found in the cells of all living things. ATP captures chemical energy obtained from the breakdown of food molecules and releases it to fuel other cellular processes.

are simple soluble sugars, like glucose, fructose, and galactose are the building blocks of disaccharides and polysaccharides. The glucose that exists in our bodies is the same glucose that exists in nature. Glucose has six carbon molecules, and the energy is stored in the carbon bonds. Our bodies extract the energy from these carbon bonds through various biomechanisms. Galactose is the sugar present in milk, and it gives sweetness to milk. Fructose is the sugar present in fruits and gives fruits their sweet taste. Fructose is also called "fruit sugar."

Monosaccharides are easy to absorb. Once we consume them, they are easily absorbed by intestinal cells and quickly taken to the liver through blood. Hence, when we consume a diet rich in monosaccharides, blood sugar levels rise, and sugar gets dumped into our liver and intestines. An abundance of sugar is a major cause of nonalcoholic fatty liver disease, which is one of the causes of obesity and diabetes. Thus, overconsumption of monosaccharides leads to several diseases.

Does that mean that we should not eat fruits? Not necessarily. Eat the whole fruit but say no to fruit juices. Along with fructose, fruits also have fiber and starch, which slows the digestion and absorption of sugar compared to drinking fruit juice loaded with fructose. To better control your blood sugar levels, consume foods with a low glycemic index (GI). Foods with a high GI are processed very quickly in our intestines and rapidly increase blood sugar. For example, eat an apple instead of drinking apple juice. Apple juice will raise your blood sugar levels immediately, but an apple will not because the apple has fiber, which is not present in apple juice. Apples have a low GI, but apple juice has a high GI. Eat a green apple instead of a red apple. Green apples are a bit tart and less sweet and have less fructose than red ones. Replace white bread with whole wheat, whole-grain, or sprouted-grain bread. Instead of eating just bread, eat a vegetable sandwich because vegetables in your sandwich have fiber, which will reduce the GI of your meal.

Disaccharides are made of two monosaccharides and are also soluble in water. Types of disaccharides are sucrose (glucose + fructose), lactose (galactose + glucose), and maltose (glucose + glucose). Disaccharides have to be broken down into their monosaccharide constituents to be absorbed into the intestine. Our body needs enzymes to break down disaccharides. Sucrose consists of two monosaccharides: glucose and fructose, and our body needs the enzyme sucrase to break down sucrose. Maltose consists of two glucose molecules, and our body needs the enzyme maltase to break it down. Lactose consists of glucose and galactose. Our bodies need lactase to break lactose down.

In my career, I have come across many people who are lactose intolerant. Lactose intolerance occurs because, for some people, the amount of the enzyme lactase decreases with age, resulting in the inability of their bodies to break down and absorb lactose.

Lactose intolerance occurs because, for some people, the amount of the enzyme lactase decreases with age, resulting in the inability of their bodies to break down and absorb lactose.

The third type of carbohydrate is the polysaccharide. These are long chains of monosaccharides and disaccharides bonded together. The common polysaccharide is starch. Foods like potatoes and white rice are examples of starches. Our bodies can easily break down starches into monosaccharides, or simple sugars, through complex metabolic processes. This is the cause of sluggishness after consuming a heavy pasta meal or lots of white rice and potatoes. Hence, it is essential to limit the intake of carbohydrates. The second type of polysaccharide, which is very important for our health because our body does not absorb it, is fiber. Fiber is a long chain of monosaccharides and disaccharides held together just like starches, but the enzymes in our body and our digestive tract cannot break them down. Thus, having fiber at every meal has its advantages and health benefits. Fiber plays a significant role in reducing the GI of the food we consume, and it helps to remove undigested food material and toxins from our gut. We shall also discuss the importance of fiber and probiotics later in the book.

As disaccharides and polysaccharides take more time to be metabolized than monosaccharides, it takes more time for the energy to be available when we consume disaccharides or polysaccharides.

The digestion of food and carbohydrates starts in the mouth. Our salivary glands have amylase in the saliva, which breaks down some of the starches into monosaccharides, which are sweet. Thus, chewing helps us break down the starches, and it is highly recommended that you chew the food properly and sit and focus on the meal when you are eating.

We learned that carbohydrates are an essential energy source, but overconsumption can lead to conditions like diabetes. It is necessary to learn about different types of carbohydrates and eat a balanced meal. At the end of the digestion process, all carbohydrates are converted into monosaccharides (simple sugar), but the time it takes for them to be converted into simple sugar depends on the type of the carbohydrate. The more complex the carbohydrate is, the longer it takes to be digested, and the more time it takes for the sugar to reach your bloodstream. That is why eating a balanced meal is essential so that you can reduce the Glycemic Index of the meal and won't have a large amount of glucose in your bloodstream.

Protein:

These days there's a lot of confusion going around regarding protein. Most people have no idea what some great sources of protein are, why they need to eat protein, and how much protein they should consume daily.

Proteins, the building blocks of our body, are made of amino acids that are linked together. Protein is used to make muscles, tendons, skin, hair, blood, connective tissues, etc. Protein also helps in making enzymes, hormones, and other body chemicals. Protein is used to build and repair tissues and helps maintain pH levels in our body, balance fluids, and boost our immune system. Protein also helps us with weight loss by increasing our metabolism and reducing our appetite, helping us feel fuller for a more extended period. Combine it with fiber to get great results. Protein and fiber also help manage our blood sugar levels by reducing the GI of the foods we consume.

Now that we've seen the importance of protein, let's get into more detail about how much protein we should consume and review some great protein sources. Due to the high-protein diet trends in the industry, we consume far more protein than we need. Yes, athletes and bodybuilders may need more protein, but most people don't need more than 10 percent of their total caloric intake to come from protein daily. Still, we often end up eating 15 percent to 20 percent protein, and if that protein is in the form of animal protein, we end up consuming a diet that is very high in saturated fat. Animal protein has more fat than plant protein, and it is often cooked using more fat.

Due to the high-protein diet trends in the industry, we consume far more protein than we need.

Research has proven that a high-fat diet is linked to heart disease, coronary artery disease, and cancer. As we read earlier, proteins are made of amino acids. Some of these amino acids are made by our body, while others are not. The latter ones are essential amino acids. As our body does not produce these, we need to include them in our diet. As animal protein provides all the nine essential amino acids, most nutrition experts recommend eating meat and dairy. I do not consume meat, and I am not a big fan of animal protein for several reasons, mainly because you will consume more fat when you consume animal protein. Also, when you consume animal protein, you consume whatever that animal ate. So, if that animal was fed antibiotics and growth hormones, you consume that unless you eat organic meat, which is free of hormones and antibiotics. This is one of the reasons for obesity, hormonal imbalance, and antibiotic resistance among meat-eaters.

When we obtain protein from plants, we do not get all the nine essential amino acids, so protein from plants is an incomplete protein. But our body needs all nine essential amino acids, so, as a solution, we should combine plant protein from two or more different sources, to get all the essential amino acids, for example, beans or lentils and brown rice, or a smoothie with nut butter, plant protein powder, and chia seeds. The combination of rice and beans will create a complete protein with all the nice essential amino acids because rice has eight amino acids out of nine, and it is low in lysine, while Beans contain isoleucine and lysine but lack methionine and tryptophan. So, when we combine rice and beans, it becomes complete protein with all nine essential amino acids.

Here are some great sources of protein for vegetarians:

- Tofu
- Edamame
- Lentils
- Chickpeas and beans

- Nuts and nut butter
- Green peas
- Seeds (chia seeds, flax seeds, sunflower seeds, pumpkin seeds, and hemp seeds)
- Buckwheat, quinoa, amaranth, farro, wheat, millet (bajra, ragi), jawar (sorghum), Jav (barley)
- Sprouts (moong bean sprouts)
- Broccoli
- Alfalfa sprouts
- Spinach
- Watercress
- Collard and mustard greens
- Greek yogurt and low-fat milk

Usually, an active adult needs 0.8 grams of protein per kilogram of body weight or 0.36 grams of protein per pound of body weight. You can also use this online protein calculator: https://www.nal.usda.gov/fnic/dri-calculator/

Just make sure you are not consuming too much protein. Use an app to maintain a diet diary to take the guesswork out.

Fats:

Fats are one of the three macronutrients in our diet, along with carbohydrates and proteins. They are significant energy sources and are essential for structural and metabolic functions. Our bodies can produce fats (except for a few essential fatty acids) from other macronutrients. For example, unused energy from carbohydrates and proteins is

Usually, an active adult needs 0.8 grams of protein per kilogram of body weight or 0.36 grams of protein per pound of body weight.

converted into fat and stored in our bodies. Dietary fats are also the carriers of some flavor and aroma ingredients, and they help dissolve and carry vitamins that are not water-soluble.

In our diet, types of fats are saturated, unsaturated, polyunsaturated, monounsaturated, and trans fats. Out of these, unsaturated, polyunsaturated, and monounsaturated fats are healthy and help lower LDL cholesterol and increase HDL cholesterol. In contrast, trans fats and saturated fats are not beneficial, as they increase LDL. To maintain your blood cholesterol and triglyceride (lipid) levels as near the normal ranges as possible, the American Diabetes Association recommends limiting the amount of saturated fats and cholesterol in our diets. Saturated fats contribute to higher LDL ("bad") cholesterol levels. The amount of saturated fats should be limited to less than 10 percent of total caloric intake, and the amount of dietary cholesterol should be limited to less than 300 mg/day. Saturated fats are not healthy, but, at the same time, they are not as harmful as trans fats.

We must limit the use of fat, and the fat we eat should be high in mono- and polyunsaturated fats. But all fat is not bad. Our bodies cannot make omega-3 fatty acids, which are polyunsaturated fats, and they are highly beneficial for our health. Omega-3s improve eye health, bone health, joint health, skin health, and brain health. Omega-3 fatty acids help reduce cardiovascular diseases, depression and anxiety, inflammation, autoimmune diseases, and Alzheimer's. They also help prevent fatty liver syndrome. Fish oil, flax seeds, walnuts, and chia seeds are high in omega-3 fatty acids.

If you studied Harvard University's Healthy Eating Plate, a guideline for a balanced meal, they recommend consuming healthy fats in moderation. Healthy fats are derived from plants, and some examples of healthy fats are avocados, avocado oil, sesame oil, olives, olive oil, nuts, and nut butter. Consume tree nuts and not ground nuts. Peanuts are groundnuts, and studies have shown that they are inflammatory, but you can consume nuts like almonds, walnuts, macadamia nuts, Brazil nuts, pistachios, cashews, pecans, pine nuts, etc. Also, sunflower seeds, sesame seeds, and pumpkin seeds are super healthy. You can also consume organic ghee.

Avoid animal fats and partially hydrogenated oils at all costs because they contain trans-fat. Choose plant oils that are rich in unsaturated fats, minimize the use of saturated fats, and say no to foods that contain animal fats (like lard), red meat (like beef), high-fat dairy, and margarine, which are packed with trans-fat.

In short, good fats are monounsaturated and polyunsaturated fats, as they lower the risk of cardiovascular diseases and other diseases. Bad fats are trans fats, as they increase the risk of cardiovascular diseases, even when eaten in small quantities.

While minimal use of saturated fats is okay, as they are not as harmful as trans fats, they also negatively impact health. Foods containing large amounts of saturated fat include red meat, butter, cheese, and ice cream. Some plant-based fats, like coconut oil and palm oil, are also rich in saturated fat. By the way, there is a simple way to identify saturated fats: They solidify quickly at colder temperatures.

These days use of coconut oil is very popular among the wellness community, but coconut oil is very controversial. Some health gurus claim that it contains MCTs (medium-chain triglycerides), which are quickly absorbed by the body, promote satiety, prevent fat storage, and are readily available for energy, but not all coconut oil contains MCTs. If you wish to consume MCTs as a fat source, you may buy MCT oil rather than commercial coconut oil because commercial coconut oil contains lauric acid, which is metabolized slowly, as are other long-chain fatty acids.

The discussion about fat would be incomplete if I did not mention ghee. You might ask: What is ghee? Butter is used in everything in the Western world, while ghee is used in India and neighboring countries. In Ayurveda, ghee is highly recommended over butter. Ghee is clarified butter, where the milk solids are removed by heating. Hence, it becomes healthier for people who are lactose intolerant. As the milk solids have been removed, ghee has a higher smoke point; therefore, it is more suitable for cooking. Cow ghee is a rich source of antioxidants and is high in anti-inflammatory properties. It is also high in monosaturated omega-3s and is a nutritional powerhouse.

Cow ghee is a rich source of antioxidants and is high in anti-inflammatory properties.

Research has shown that there is a link between the consumption of animal protein, trans fat, saturated fat, and cardiovascular diseases, as well as cancer. Also, high fat consumption is directly associated with cancer because of bile. Bile juice produced by our liver is necessary for the absorption of fat. The more fat you eat, the more bile is produced to absorb it. Bile is a carcinogen. So, the more fat you eat, the more carcinogen you make. Colon cancer, breast cancer, and prostate cancer are mainly influenced by the amount of fat we eat. Hence, I am not a fan of ketogenic diets.

Thus, fat should not be a significant source of energy in our diet, as our bodies do convert unused energy gained from carbohydrates and proteins into fat for storage purposes, but we do need to consume a small amount of fat because some vitamins, like vitamin A, D, E, and K, are fat-soluble. These vitamins play a crucial role in our well-being. Vitamin A plays a vital role in maintaining healthy vision, a healthy immune system, cellular growth, hair growth, and reproductive health. Vitamin D, also called the "sunshine vitamin," is responsible for bone and immune health. Vitamin E is a powerful antioxidant and natural blood thinner. It protects your cells from premature aging, oxidative damage, and muscle weakness. Vitamin K is vital for blood clotting and supports bone health. In our next chapter, we will learn more about all the vitamins and micronutrients.

References:

- Alberts B, Johnson A, Lewis J, et al. Molecular Biology of the Cell. 4th edition. New York: Garland Science; 2002. How Cells Obtain Energy from Food. Available from: https://www.ncbi.nlm.nih.gov/books/NBK26882/

- National Institute on Aging. 2021. Important Nutrients to Know: Proteins, Carbohydrates, and Fats. [online] Available at: https://www.nia.nih.gov/health/important-nutrients-know-proteins-carbohydrates-and-fats

- National Research Council (US) Committee on Diet and Health. Diet and Health: Implications for Reducing Chronic Disease Risk. Washington (DC): National Academies Press (US); 1989. 8, Protein. Available from: https://www.ncbi.nlm.nih.gov/books/NBK218739/

- Rix I, Nexøe-Larsen C, Bergmann NC, et al. Glucagon Physiology. [Updated 2019 Jul 16]. In: Feingold KR, Anawalt B, Boyce A, et al., editors. Endotext [Internet]. South Dartmouth (MA): MDText.com, Inc.; 2000-. Available from: https://www.ncbi.nlm.nih.gov/books/NBK279127/

- National Research Council (US) Committee on Diet and Health. Diet and Health: Implications for Reducing Chronic Disease Risk. Washington (DC): National Academies Press (US); 1989. 9, Carbohydrates. Available from: https://www.ncbi.nlm.nih.gov/books/NBK218753/

- *National Research Council (US) Committee on Diet and Health. Diet and Health: Implications for Reducing Chronic Disease Risk. Washington (DC): National Academies Press (US); 1989. 7, Fats and Other Lipids. Available from: https://www.ncbi.nlm.nih.gov/books/ NBK218759/*

- *Sankararaman S, Sferra TJ. Are We Going Nuts on Coconut Oil? Curr Nutr Rep. 2018 Sep;7(3):107–115. doi: 10.1007/s13668-018-0230-5. PMID: 29974400. Available from: https://pubmed.ncbi.nlm.nih.gov/29974400/*

- *Mathes P, Thiery J. Die Rolle des Lipidstoffwechsels in der Prävention der koronaren Herzerkrankung [The role of lipid metabolism in the prevention of coronary heart disease]. Z Kardiol. 2005;94 Suppl 3:III/43–55. German. doi: 10.1007/s00392-005-1307-x. PMID: 16258792. Available from: https://pubmed.ncbi.nlm.nih.gov/16258792/*

- *St-Onge MP, Bosarge A. Weight-loss diet that includes consumption of medium-chain triacylglycerol oil leads to a greater rate of weight and fat mass loss than does olive oil. Am J Clin Nutr. 2008 Mar;87(3):621–6. doi: 10.1093/ajcn/87.3.621. PMID: 18326600; PMCID: PMC2874190. Available from: https://pubmed.ncbi.nlm.nih.gov/18326600/*

- *St-Onge, M. P., Mayrsohn, B., O'Keeffe, M., Kissileff, H. R., Choudhury, A. R., & Laferrère, B. (2014). Impact of medium and long-chain triglycerides consumption on appetite and food intake in overweight men. European journal of clinical nutrition, 68(10), 1134–1140. https://doi.org/10.1038/ejcn.2014.145 Available from: https://www.ncbi.nlm.nih.gov/pmc/articles/PMC4192077/*

CHAPTER 8

Micronutrients

As per the World Health Organization, micronutrients are vitamins and trace minerals needed by the body in minute amounts. However, their impact on a body's health is critical, and deficiency in any of them can cause severe and even life-threatening conditions. They perform various functions, including enabling the body to produce enzymes, hormones, and other substances needed for normal growth and development.

Micronutrients are the group of nutrients consisting of vitamins and minerals required by our body to perform several metabolic functions.

Micronutrients are the group of nutrients consisting of vitamins and minerals required by our body to perform several metabolic functions. They support growth, immune function, bone health, brain functions, heart health, fluid balance, energy production, and several other functions. Our body requires these essential nutrients in smaller amounts than macronutrients.

When we eat, we consume vitamins and minerals created or absorbed by plants and animals. As the micronutrient content of each food is different, it is essential to consume a variety of foods. That is why experts recommend we eat fruits and vegetables of all colors.

Most vitamins are water-soluble, and they are flushed out of our bodies when consumed in excess. We will not go into detail about all vitamins and minerals, but we shall discuss a few main vitamins and minerals.

Water-soluble Vitamins:

- **Vitamin B1 (thiamine):** Converts nutrients from our food into energy.
- **Vitamin B2 (riboflavin):** Helps in energy production, cell function, and fat metabolism.
- **Vitamin B3 (niacin):** Helps in energy production from our food.
- **Vitamin B5 (pantothenic acid):** Helps in fatty acid synthesis.
- **Vitamin B6 (pyridoxine):** Helps to convert stored carbohydrates to sugar for energy production and helps in the creation of new red blood cells.
- **Vitamin B7 (biotin):** Plays a vital role in the metabolism of fatty acids, amino acids, and glucose.
- **Vitamin B9 (folate):** Helps in cell division.
- **Vitamin B12 (cobalamin):** Aids proper brain function and production of red blood cells.
- **Vitamin C (ascorbic acid):** Potent antioxidant. Helps improve immune function, biosynthesis of collagen, and protein metabolism.

As these vitamins are not stored in our body, nor can we produce them, it is essential to take them regularly, either through the food we eat or through supplementation.

Fat-soluble Vitamins:

Fat-soluble vitamins do not dissolve in water, and they are best absorbed when taken along with fat. Also, they are stored in our liver or fatty tissues for future use. It is crucial that you only consume these vitamins if your doctor or a professional recommends them. The names and functions of fat-soluble vitamins are:

- **Vitamin A:** Helps in improving vision and organ function.
- **Vitamin D:** Helps immune function. It also helps with calcium absorption and bone growth.
- **Vitamin E:** Powerful antioxidant. Protects cells from damage and aids in immune function.
- **Vitamin K:** Helps with bone development and blood clotting.

Trace minerals:

Here are some of the minerals required by our body in trace amounts:

- **Calcium:** Necessary for healthy bones and teeth. It also helps with muscle function.
- **Phosphorus:** Necessary for healthy bones; it also forms cell membranes.
- **Magnesium:** Helps in enzyme reactions and in regulating blood pressure.
- **Sodium:** An electrolyte that maintains fluid balance and blood pressure.
- **Chloride:** Helps maintain fluid balance.
- **Potassium:** Helps maintain fluid balance in cells and with nerve transmission and muscle function.

- **Sulfur:** Important component of our tissues and amino acids like methionine and cysteine.
- **Iron:** Helps provide oxygen to our muscles and aids in creating certain hormones.
- **Copper:** Required for normal brain and nervous system function.
- **Zinc:** Required for healthy immune function, growth, and healing of wounds.
- **Iodine:** Helps regulate the thyroid. Required for healthy growth of fetus and infants. Required for cognitive development.
- **Fluoride:** Helps in bone and teeth development.
- **Selenium:** Assists in maintaining thyroid health, reproductive health and protects against oxidative damage.
- **Chromium picolinate:** Improves glucose metabolism, helps reduce body fat, and increases lean muscle mass.

References:

- *World Health Organization. (n.d.). Micronutrients. World Health Organization. https://www.who.int/health-topics/micronutrients#tab=tab_1.*
- *Shenkin A. Micronutrients in health and disease. Postgrad Med J. 2006 Sep;82(971):559-67. doi: 10.1136/pgmj.2006.047670. PMID: 16954450; PMCID: PMC2585731. Available from: https://www.ncbi.nlm.nih.gov/pmc/articles/PMC2585731/*
- *Centers for Disease Control and Prevention. (2020, December 3). Micronutrient Facts. Centers for Disease Control and Prevention. https://www.cdc.gov/nutrition/micronutrient-malnutrition/micronutrients/index.html.*

CHAPTER 9

Role of Probiotics and Fiber

A t the time of birth, our body is sterile, free of microorganisms, but within hours of birth, our body and gastrointestinal (GI) tract become host to microbial colonies. Within a few days of birth, microbial colonies start to establish in our GI tract, and mother's milk helps good bacteria colonize while keeping bad ones at bay. Thus, mother's milk is essential, especially colostrum, as it supports a good microbiome while protecting us from harmful ones.

Our human body is host to millions and millions of microbiomes. According to research, microbes outnumber human cells in our bodies. Several research studies are being conducted to understand the impact of these microbes on our food cravings, health, digestion, immunity, obesity, and mood. For more information, you can study the Human Microbiome Project launched by the National Institute of Health (NIH) at www.hmpdacc.org.

Several studies have proven preliminary evidence that gut bacteria have a beneficial effect on your immunity, digestion, mood, and anxiety, partly by affecting the activity of your vagus nerve. The more diverse and more affluent the microbial colonies, the better is our health. Low diversity means you will be more prone to obesity, high cholesterol, insulin resistance, weakened immune system, polycystic ovary syndrome (PCOS), allergies, inflammation, diabetes, etc. While good microbes aid in food digestion, bad ones cause indigestion, creating toxins, leading to ill health. While good microbes can enhance our health, the bad ones can cause deterioration.

Probiotics are live microorganisms that are safe to consume and can help improve our overall health and immunity. They help with food digestion, the production of compounds to destroy the harmful microbes, and help maintain the pH of your gut. Now, it is difficult to digest—no pun intended—that the microorganisms are good for us because, in today's world, we are used to believing that to be healthy, we must be germ-free. We believe this to such an extent that people develop germaphobia, but the truth is that not all microbes are harmful.

Probiotics are live microorganisms that are safe to consume and can help improve our overall health and immunity.

There is a symbiotic mutualism relationship between our gut microbiome and us. The DNA of these trillions of gut bacteria is woven into our DNA. These trillions of bacteria support our life by supporting our health and immune system. Hence the researchers quote that our immune system resides in our gut. The microbes in our gut help with our sleep, stress response, and ability to fight several illnesses.

At the same time, not all microbes are good for us, and there is a constant fight between our friends and foes within our bodies. Hence, we must live a lifestyle to maintain the balance of good microbes.

We help our friends so that they can help us. We must learn to feed the good microbes to have rich and diverse microbial colonies in our body, which will help us fight harmful disease-causing microbes, like Candida and E. coli (toxic strains) *Staphylococcus*.

Over-use of alcohol or substance abuse; stress; excessive consumption of sugar, high-fructose corn syrup, and artificial sweeteners; high-fat diets; meat; sugar; chlorine and fluoride in drinking water; antibiotics; processed food filled with additives, preservatives, and chemicals; exposure to environmental toxins; and many other factors could change the balance of our intestinal flora. In short, the modern Western diet low in fiber and high in sugar, salt, fat, and processed food is harmful to our gut microbiome.

Now, you might question, how do we accomplish the goal of having diverse microbial colonies in our body, as well as in our GI tract? The answer is simple. There is a direct link between the food we eat and the biodiversity in our gut. Hence, providing an environment for these gut microbes to flourish through the right diet, good sleep, and proper lifestyle habits makes sense. The beneficial bacteria in your gut feed on the undigested food, i.e., fiber and complex starches. Thus, the food we consume is not only the energy source for us but also helps our gut bacteria thrive. So, it is essential for us to switch from a traditional American diet that is low in fiber and high in fat and sugar to a diet that is rich in fiber. Consume whole grains, legumes, fruits, leafy green vegetables, root vegetables, nuts, and seeds as these foods are high in fiber and complex starch.

If you consume sugar, you will have microbes that thrive on the sugar in your gut. These microbes are harmful to us, as they cause damage to our gut lining, as well as inflammation. Thus, the food we eat will change our gut microbiome, eventually changing the course of our health.

Live a lifestyle that supports you and these friends of yours while avoiding things that will help the harmful disease-causing bacteria flourish. When you eat something, remember that your food can either feed the healthy microbiomes or the harmful ones.

Research has yet to give an accurate definition of a normal gut microbiome, but it has proven a direct correlation between a healthy diet and rich, diverse microbial colonies in our body, as well as the GI tract.

To support diverse microbial colonies, you can follow some of these mindful eating tips, which we shall discuss in detail in our later chapters:

- Eliminate foods that cause or increase low-level chronic inflammation, like sugar and processed foods, filled with colors, artificial flavors, and preservatives.
- Eliminate red meat, saturated and trans fats, refined sugar, high-fructose corn syrup, refined flour, white rice, groundnuts, sugary sodas, artificial sweeteners, and foods containing antibiotics and hormones.
- Eat what grows on plants, not those made in plants.
- Eat whole grains, healthy fats (like olive oil, organic dairy, ghee, and tree nuts), and seeds (like chia, pumpkin, and sunflower).
- Eat foods that are rich in probiotics to nourish your gut. Foods like kimchi, yogurt, kefir, kombucha, and other fermented food.
- Consume plenty of prebiotics, like soluble and insoluble fiber, to feed your gut microbiome. Fiber is an excellent source of nutrition for microbes. Fruits, leafy green vegetables, and whole grains are excellent fiber sources.

Also, the most important thing to speculate is that not all probiotic supplements are made the same. These days, people have become health-conscious, and they take probiotic supplements. There is nothing wrong with this as long as you pick the right source, as health benefits from probiotic supplements are strain-specific, and not all strains are helpful. Some companies make claims on their nutrition label, which have been proven false in laboratory testing. Just taking probiotic supplements from one strain is not going to benefit much. One should take a supplement that gives you a variety of strains. You can do some research on NIH.com, read reviews about the brand, learn to understand nutrition labels, and pick the brand whose label lists multiple strains of the microbiome in your probiotics. To learn more about probiotics, feel free to visit *https://www.ncbi.nlm.nih.gov/pmc/articles/PMC2995750/*.

Moreover, try to get a supplement with naturally strong strains to withstand harsh stomach conditions and arrive in the gut alive. The strains should also have the natural ability to adhere to the gut and grow, or else you are flushing your money down the drain. My personal favorite is Nutrilite™ Balance Within™ Probiotic, as a single serving contains 6.3 billion colony-forming units (CFU) of clinically tested beneficial live probiotic microorganisms from five different strains. It is also powered by patented arrive-alive technology, which has naturally strong strains that can resist the harsh conditions of the stomach to arrive in the gut alive. It also has patented stick-to-gut technology that gives a natural ability to adhere to the gut, helping to promote a balance of good bacteria with daily use. It also contains prebiotic fiber inulin to encourage the growth of healthy gut flora when taken with a diet rich in fiber.

Now, the question is why fiber is so essential to our diet. Every health article emphasizes consuming dietary fiber. What is fiber? Fiber is a type of carbohydrate that our body cannot digest, and it is present in fruits, vegetables, and whole grains. While most carbohydrates are broken down into simple sugar, fiber will not be broken down into sugar, and it will pass through the body undigested.

In layman's terms, dietary fiber is like a cleaning brush, which will scrub the undigested food and toxins from your gastrointestinal tract when it passes through the body. It plays a vital role in maintaining a healthy gastrointestinal tract, and, hence, every meal should be a balanced meal, including fiber. There are two types of fiber: soluble and insoluble. Both have a specific role in the digestion process, and both are equally important. Soluble fiber dissolves in water and is a source of food for good gut bacteria, while insoluble fiber can soak up water in the intestine, giving you a feeling of fullness to curb appetite. Whole grains, fruits, vegetables, beans and legumes, nuts, and seeds have high fiber content.

In layman's terms, dietary fiber is like a cleaning brush, which will scrub the undigested food and toxins from your gastrointestinal tract when it passes through the body.

Processed foods like eggs, meat, and dairy have low or no fiber content. That's why it is essential to have a balanced meal. For example, switch to wheat bread from white bread. Add a few vegetables, like cucumber, carrots, and lettuce, to your bread, and eat it as a sandwich instead of eating your bread with sugary jams.

If you are eating out and wheat pasta is not available, you can eat white pasta, but add protein and vegetables to your pasta. Also, add a salad to your plate to bring back the balance in your meal. Eat a fruit or a couple of dates instead of drinking fruit juice, soda, or eating sugary desserts. When we add fiber to our diet, it reduces the glycemic index (GI) of the food we consume. A low GI diet aids in balancing blood sugar levels. Over and above that, fiber helps prevent constipation, balances blood sugar, helps decrease bad cholesterol, and curbs appetite.

At the same time, it is essential to maintain balance and not consume too much fiber because excess fiber can cause diarrhea and bloating. It is recommended that men should consume 38 grams of fiber, and women should consume 25 grams of fiber daily in their diet. Anything in excess is not good.

It is advisable to maintain a diet diary to be mindful of what you are eating. Also, nowadays, there are many apps available that can help us retain a diet diary and calculate the macronutrients in our diet.

References:

- *Amara AA, Shibl A. Role of Probiotics in health improvement, infection control, and disease treatment and management. Saudi Pharm J. 2015 Apr;23(2):107-14. doi: 10.1016/j.jsps.2013.07.001. Epub 2013 Jul 18. PMID: 25972729; PMCID: PMC4421088. Available from: https://www.ncbi.nlm.nih.gov/pmc/articles/PMC4421088/*
- *Zhang YJ, Li S, Gan RY, Zhou T, Xu DP, Li HB. Impacts of gut bacteria on human health and diseases. Int J Mol Sci. 2015 Apr 2;16(4):7493-519. doi: 10.3390/ijms16047493. PMID: 25849657; PMCID: PMC4425030. Available from: https://www.ncbi.nlm.nih.gov/pmc/articles/PMC4425030/*
- *U.S. Department of Health and Human Services. (n.d.). Probiotics: What you need to know. National Center for Complementary and Integrative Health. Retrieved November 30, 2021, from https://www.nccih.nih.gov/health/probiotics-what-you-need-to-know.*

CHAPTER 10

Digestive Fire A.K.A Metabolism

꧁꧂

As per conventional medicine, digestion is a complex process that involves transformation of the food we intake into nutrients and the elimination of waste material. The digestion of food begins in our mouth when we chew and swallow, but the majority of it occurs in our gastrointestinal tract utilizing various enzymes, stomach acids, bile, and hormones. The organs that are part of our gastrointestinal tract are the mouth, esophagus, stomach, small intestine, large intestine, rectum, anus, liver, pancreas, and gall bladder. Over and above that, your gut microbiome plays a vital role in the digestion process. Once the food is digested, the nutrients are carried via the circulatory system to various parts of your body, and the waste is eliminated through the anus. Along with your gastrointestinal tract, the central nervous system plays an important role in digestion by secreting hormones, enzymes, and digestive juices responsible for digestion and also by sending signals to control the actions of contraction and relaxation in your gut muscles so that the food can reach your small intestine. Metabolism refers to how the cells in your body utilize the energy and nutrients they obtain from food through digestion.

In Ayurveda, the term "Agni" is used for both digestion and metabolism. Agni means fire, and fire has the capability to transform anything it comes in contact with. Ingested food is digested, absorbed, and assimilated, which is a critical function for the maintenance of life and is performed by agni. According to ancient Ayurvedic texts, there are 13 types of agni, but in this chapter, we will only talk about your digestive fire, which is called *Jatharagni* in Sanskrit, and it is the most important, as it digests the food and transforms it into vitality. As per Ayurveda, there are

> *Agni means fire, and fire has the capability to transform anything it comes in contact with.*

four types of jatharagni; balanced, irregular, sharp, and weak. The function of your digestive fire or jatharagni is to transform the food you eat into energy required for all the functions of your body. When your digestive fire is balanced and robust, you will lead a long, happy, healthy life, as it will transform the food you ingest into ojas (vitality) but if the digestive fire is irregular or weakened, it will

> *As per Ayurveda, there are four types of jatharagni; balanced, irregular, sharp, and weak.*

create ama that builds up as toxins and is transported to various organs of your body through your circulatory system, resulting in chronic inflammation that causes ill health or disease. These toxins are nothing but residues of undigested food that rots in your gut due to weak digestive fire. Hence the digestive fire is the foundation of life, and it is vital to have a balanced digestive fire so that we can easily metabolize our food, to produce all the nutrients required for healthy cells, muscles, tissues, and bones. On an emotional level, a balanced agni helps us to process and respond to all the experiences in a healthy manner.

These toxins are nothing but residues of undigested food that rots in your gut due to weak digestive fire.

Thus, our health depends on how healthy our digestive fire is, and the health of our digestive fire depends on the food we eat and drink, as well as our environment. When someone's digestive fire is weak, they will feel heavy, sluggish, sleepy, and fatigued all the time, especially after meals. They lack energy and zest for life. If someone's digestive fire is very sharp, they are prone to hyperacidity, heartburn, and acid reflux. In short, when your agni is not balanced, you may get ill frequently due to a compromised immune system and become host to chronic diseases and conditions, like diabetes, high blood pressure, migraines, arthritis, leaky gut syndrome, acid reflux, obesity, celiac disease, Crohn's disease, irritable bowel syndrome, gas, bloating, burping, constipation, water retention, heart diseases, and a lot more. Every disease starts with poor digestion.

Here are a few symptoms of poor digestion. Signs that you have lost the fire in your belly:

- Feeling sleepy and sluggish after meals
- Having the urge to poop right after eating meals
- Gas and bloating
- Fatigue, lack of energy, and zest
- Lack of appetite or reduced appetite
- Poor immune system

- Irritable bowel syndrome, gas, bloating, burping, constipation
- Lack of sleep or sleep disturbances and waking up tired.
- Migraines, upset stomach, allergies
- Chronic inflammation and autoimmune diseases
- Unintentional weight changes

Imagine your digestive fire as a wood-burning fireplace. If you want a robust and steady fire in the fireplace, you will not add anything that will extinguish the fire, right? The same principle is true for your digestive fire.

While we explained in this chapter the importance of having a robust digestive fire, in later chapters, we shall touch upon some tips on how to keep your digestive fire burning strong.

References:

- *Chopra, D. D., Kshirsagar, D. S., Simon, D. D., Patel, D. S., Porter, D. V., Saint, D. M., Gabriel, R., Stern, E., & Nadarajah, M. (2019, November). The perfect health ayurvedic lifestyle online enrichment program. Session 1 - 15.*
- *Agrawal, A. K., Yadav, C. R., & Meena, M. S. (2010). Physiological aspects of Agni. Ayu, 31(3), 395–398. https://www.ncbi.nlm.nih.gov/pmc/articles/PMC3221079/*
- *U.S. Department of Health and Human Services. (n.d.). Your digestive system & how it works. National Institute of Diabetes and Digestive and Kidney Diseases. Retrieved February 10, 2022, from https://www.niddk.nih.gov/health-information/digestive-diseases/digestive-system-how-it-works*

CHAPTER 11

Dosha, or Our Unique Mind-Body Constitution

❦

Ayurveda is the world's most sophisticated mind-body health system, developed thousands of years before modern medicine by the sages of India. Ayurveda is the science of life. Instead of just treating symptoms of illness, it addresses the root cause of the illness. It focuses on improving the health of mind, body, spirit, and environment so we can experience our fullest potential by achieving a state of optimal well-being.

As per Ayurveda, each human being has a unique physical, physiological, and mental constitution, and hence each human being is unique, and when they have a disease, they require a correspondingly unique treatment regime. To understand all this, one must first understand the basic Ayurvedic principles. In Ayurvedic philosophy, three doshas—vata, pitta, and kapha—determine an individual's unique combination of physical, physiological, and psychological features. The prakriti of a person—prakriti is a Sanskrit word for nature—is based on the relative proportions of the three doshas.

Dosha, which means "unique mind-body constitution," is the foundation of Ayurveda. It is essential to learn about our unique mind-body constitution to understand ourselves, our personalities, strengths, and weaknesses. Also, it helps us to understand others. Most importantly, we can figure out what type of diet and exercise is good for our well-being and what is not so good. It helps us make daily choices for our optimal well-being, and it's fun learning about your dosha.

Dosha, which means "unique mind-body constitution," is the foundation of Ayurveda.

To understand the dosha, you must first understand five elements, also called Pancha mahabhutas in Sanskrit, where Pancha means "five," and mahabhutas mean "elements." These are the building blocks of the universe, and everything in our physical universe, including our body, comprises these five elements:

- Space (akasha) – pure potential and infinite possibilities
- Air (vayu) – movement and change
- Fire (tejas) – transformation and creativity
- Water (jala) – cohesion and lubrication
- Earth (prithvi) – structure and stability

These five elements combine into three primary patterns called doshas:

- Vata dosha (ectomorph): space + air
- Pitta dosha (mesomorph): fire + water
- Kapha dosha (endomorph): water + earth

We all have all three doshas in our individual mind-body constitution, but the proportion of these doshas will vary from person to person. Your unique balance of vata, pitta, and kapha dosha will determine your unique mind-body constitution, or your basic prakriti, the Sanskrit word for nature. Most people have one predominant dosha, which will be their primary dosha, and then other secondary doshas. For example, a particular individual's pitta may be their primary dosha and kapha their secondary dosha. Hence, this individual would be referred to as the pitta kapha type.

Your dosha, or prakriti, is determined at the time of conception, and it remains the same throughout your life. When these doshas are in balance or harmony, our mind and body are in the state of optimal well-being, but, during our life, due to the choices we make, our doshas can become imbalanced. This is when we experience illness or disease. The disease is nothing but the absence of ease. The state in which our doshas are out of balance is called vikriti, which means we are in a state of imbalance.

Your dosha, or prakriti, is determined at the time of conception, and it remains the same throughout your life.

When your doshas are in balance, you are in an optimal state of well-being. Whatever your intake may be through your five senses, including food, water, other fluids, and experiences, gets metabolized efficiently and converted into ojas, the Sanskrit word for vitality. When your doshas are not in balance, whatever you intake through your five senses gets converted into ama, which is the Sanskrit term for toxins. When these toxins build up in our body at a cellular level, we experience chronic inflammation.

Under normal conditions, our body has the miraculous ability to stay in a state of optimal well-being by flushing out toxins and repairing itself on a daily basis. But we get in its way by making poor lifestyle choices. When our doshas are totally out of balance, the amount of toxins generated is greater than our body's ability to flush them out, and they start building up and getting stored at a cellular level, causing chronic inflammation. Also, these toxins find weak spots in our body and start accumulating there to cause localized chronic inflammation, resulting in lifestyle-related illnesses and conditions, like diabetes, high blood pressure, coronary artery disease, autoimmune disorders, arthritis, obesity, insomnia, allergies, and many more.

Hence, it is super important to understand your dosha to make daily choices that will keep your dosha in balance and you in a state of optimal well-being. So let us discuss each dosha in detail, including the qualities of the dosha, as well as what happens when the dosha is out of balance. We shall also briefly discuss the do's and don'ts of staying in balance.

Vibrant Vata (Ectomorph): Movement and Agility

As vata is made of space and air elements, this dosha is about movement. Vata controls all the movement in the body. It controls the flow of blood, the flow of lymphatic fluid, vocal cords when you speak, the motion of body parts like arms and legs, and even the movement and speed of thoughts.

Qualities of Vata: Qualities of vata are the same as qualities of its elements, which are cold, light, dry, irregular, rough, moving, quick, changeable.

Here are the physical characteristics of people who have vata dosha predominance.

Physical Characteristics: Thin, light frame, agile, fast, quick, and highly mobile. They are like the squirrels of the human world.

I observe squirrels in the woods in my backyard. They are always moving. Just can't sit still. If you pay attention to nature, you will find a lot of vata creatures, like squirrels, hummingbirds, deer, rabbits, gazelle, and the cheetah. Humans who have vata dosha predominance have dry skin and hair. Their feet and legs are always cold. They are very light sleepers and have irregular and sensitive digestion. Also, they experience bursts of energy. Sometimes they feel highly energetic and get everything done in minutes, but very soon get tired and experience fatigue, as they have high speed but low endurance. Also, when it comes to eating, they tend to be nibblers. Instead of three proper meals a day, they prefer to munch and have smaller meals more frequently.

Emotional Characteristics: Vatas love excitement and new experiences. They will always be ready to start new projects but have short attention spans, so they will move on to the next exciting project before completing the previous one. They have a lot of unfinished projects in their garage. They tend to start everything quickly but finish nothing. If you go to a party, you will be able to spot vatas easily. They are starry-eyed, drawing attention, and talking with excitement with someone, and, within a couple of seconds, they are gone to share their excitement with another person, leaving the first person wondering what happened. They are very talkative and like to tell exciting, juicy stories and exaggerate things. They are quick to anger but also quick to forgive. When vatas are in balance, they are energetic, creative, artistic, and flexible. They also take the initiative and are lively conversationalists.

As we saw earlier, vatas dislike routine, so they quickly get bored. But this habit of seeking constant excitement can put them out of balance and decrease their productivity because, to succeed in anything, one must have the ability to focus and put in consistent and persistent work every single day.

For example, to get a six-pack, one must go to the gym every day and work out consistently. Failure to do so will result in failure to achieve the desired result. That is true for anything worthwhile in life. Hence, vatas must always keep their goals in front of them. Suggestions include preparing a dream board or a vision board. Staying focused on the prize will motivate the vatas to pay the price.

Also, try to bring some variety to the work if required, but don't chase every single project. Resolve to complete whatever you start. When the vata dosha becomes unbalanced, this imbalance manifests in the body as weight loss, constipation, hypertension, arthritis, weakness, restlessness, and digestive challenges. Also, when unbalanced, they worry, become anxious, and suffer from insomnia. They feel overwhelmed or stressed easily, and when they do, are likely to ask, "What did *I* do wrong?"

According to Ayurveda, our mind-body type is determined at the moment of conception. We are all born with a unique combination of the vata, pitta, and kapha doshas, which stay constant throughout our lives. This is known as our *"prakriti"* or "nature" or "the first creation." Trying to change your prakriti is like changing your height from short to tall or changing the color of your eyes from brown to blue.

Your unique mind-body constitution or dosha prakriti is the reference point, and, based on it, there will be some things that will keep you in harmony with your nature, while other things might create disharmony and cause you to move out of balance and create disease.

There is another term that one must understand: vikriti. It is your current state of imbalance, and it can change throughout the year and your lifetime. Your vikriti is influenced by your lifestyle, experiences, and choices. For example, your prakriti, or mind-body constitution, may be pitta, but if you've been busy due to work (pitta tend to become workaholics), you may not eat proper meals or get enough sleep. You start skipping meals, experiencing mental strain due to work pressure, and sleeping poorly, so you may develop a vata imbalance. We refer to this imbalance as "excess vata" or "aggravated vata."

Before we go into details on how to bring any dosha into balance, we must also understand the fundamental principle of *similarity* and *difference*. There is a fundamental principle in Ayurveda, known as the principle of *samanya* (similarity) and *vishesha* (difference). This principle of *samanya* and *vishesha* states that similarity of all substances is always the cause of the increase, and dissimilarity is the cause of the decrease. Both have an impact on their application.

This Ayurvedic principle of the same and opposite is a universal truth and is applicable, not only in balancing the doshas but everywhere in life. For example, if someone is cold and consumes cold foods or ice-cold drinks, the cold will increase, but if they consume warm foods, which create heat in the body, their cold will reduce. When someone has financial challenges and if they are consumed with thoughts about their financial challenges, their challenges will increase, but if they are consumed with thoughts about abundance and wealth, their challenges will decrease. When someone has problems in life and is consumed with thoughts about their problems, their problems will grow, but if they start focusing on solutions and become consumed with thoughts about solutions, the problems will reduce as they find solutions to their problems.

In simple terms, this principle states that equality will increase, and the opposite will decrease, so to balance overactive or out-of-balance vata, the person will need to bring in things whose qualities are opposite of the basic qualities of vata.

Ayurveda uses five senses to bring any imbalance into balance. Taste, touch, sound, sight, and smell. Sound, sight, and smell help to balance the out-of-balance vata *mind*, while taste and touch help balance the out-of-balance vata body.

Balancing Vata:

Balancing by Taste: The best tastes to pacify vata are sweet, salty, and sour. Minimize foods that are pungent, bitter, or astringent since these tastes increase vata. To counterbalance the light, dry, cool nature of the vata dosha, Ayurveda traditionally recommends foods that are heavy, oily, and warm.

Balancing by Touch: To balance vata by touch, perform massage with light, gentle strokes, with heavier, warming oils, such as sesame or almond oil.

Balancing by Sound: To balance the unbalanced vata mind, choose sounds that are warm, relaxing, slow, and grounding, such as cello compositions or Gregorian chants, or traditional classical instrumental music. Music that incorporates slow drumbeats or a steady low bass can be incredibly soothing.

Balancing by Sight: An out-of-balance vata's mind can be balanced with soft pastel colors, colors of nature, earthy tones.

Balancing by Smell: Floral, fruity, sweet, and sour aromas, such as basil, orange, geranium, clove, lavender, vanilla, and patchouli can help balance the vata mind.

Also, as we all know, it is essential to maintain a healthy exercise routine; no matter what your dosha is, knowing your dosha type is essential because you can pick the exercise that will work best with your dosha. We shall review the types of exercises that can benefit people with vata dosha dominance in Part II.

When anxious, vata types tend to eat their anxiety, and they tend to become emotional eaters. As they already have a delicate and irregular digestive fire and eating meals when anxious weakens it more. It is not recommended to eat your meals when you are emotionally upset or unstable because that's when your sympathetic nervous system is active.

We learned what happens when the sympathetic nervous system is active in the previous chapter. When you are in fight or flight mode, blood rushes to your large muscle groups, heartbeats increase, breathing is rapid, and digestion stops. At this time, your digestion is weak, and the body cannot digest food properly and produces ama (toxins) from the food you consume. Toxins are gross, heavy, sticky, and cold in properties, and they start building up in the tissues and organs. This leads to kapha imbalances in the body, as well as diseases. This shows that, no matter what your prakriti or unique mind-body constitution is, you can have an imbalance in any dosha. Someone who is vata type can have a kapha imbalance, as per the above-mentioned scenario, but, at the same time, the vata type is more prone to have vata imbalance than kapha imbalance. One more thing we need to understand is that one imbalance will lead to another, and, eventually, all the doshas can be out-of-balance.

Most of the time, the imbalance happens in the mind first and then manifests in the body. The key is to be very mindful and listen to our bodies. If you pay attention to the whispers, you will never have to address the screams. The information provided here can be overwhelming, so use the grocery store approach. Take what works for you, implement it, and leave the rest, as not everything is for everyone. In short, avoid cold temperatures and stale cold, frozen, raw food. Stay calm, stay warm, consume warm meals with healthy fats, and maintain a daily routine.

In short, avoid cold temperatures and stale cold, frozen, raw food. Stay calm, stay warm, consume warm meals with healthy fats, and maintain a daily routine.

Vibrant Vata is thy name
Creativity and agility are thy fame
Oh! Without you, the world is boring and dull
Just stay grounded to add poise and lull

Earth and Sunshine are your best friend
On meditation, you want to depend
Gives you the balance and warmth
To find your peace and true north

Be careful in cold and dry weather
Bundle up with jackets of wool and leather
Say no to capris and tees
Consume warm meals with lots of ghee

While speed and excitement are your strength
Be consistent and persistent for a length
To stay focused in the game
For the prize, you want to claim

Pastel greens and ocean hues
Will keep at bay your winter blues
Soothing jazz and calming flute
Will help you stand firm in your boots

Kruti Thakore

Passionate Pitta (Mesomorph): Transformation and metabolism

The fundamental function of pitta is transformation and metabolism. Fire and water are the elements of pitta. All bodily functions related to transformation and metabolism, like digestion of food into energy, are governed by pitta. It also governs the absorption of nutrients and body temperature.

This summer, I had the privilege of enjoying the wildlife in my backyard, and I saw a sparrow hawk. It was sitting on the fence near the bird feeder and, I guess, waiting for prey. I had never seen this bird in my backyard before, so I enjoyed this rare sight and observed how focused the bird was, patiently waiting for a couple of minutes. I realized that's my example of a pitta bird. Some other examples of pitta animals are the lion, tiger, and eagle.

Qualities of Pitta: Very similar to those of fire. Hot, light, intense, penetrating, pungent, sharp, acidic. People with a predominance of the pitta dosha have an aggressive nature, are very passionate, highly intellectual, and are born leaders. At a party or an office environment, you will spot them easily. They take charge, talking to people passionately, sharing their ideas, and leading others to follow them. When they talk, others listen and follow.

Physical Characteristics: Pitta types are usually medium-sized and weight, with bright red or brown hair and a penetrating gaze. Early graying of hair is very common. Also, baldness or thinning hair is a common problem. They are like the goats of the human world, as they have excellent digestion and, when hungry, they become angry. They sleep soundly for short periods and have a strong sex drive. When in balance, pittas have a lustrous copper-toned complexion, perfect digestion, abundant energy, and a strong appetite. They perspire easily and have warm hands and feet. When out of balance, pittas may suffer from skin rashes, burning sensations, peptic ulcers, excessive body heat, conjunctivitis, prickly heat, heartburn, and indigestion.

Emotional Characteristics: Great concentration, sharp intellect, and fantastic focus. When they're in balance, they are good decision-makers, teachers, leaders, and speakers. They are precise, blunt, sharp-witted, direct, courageous, and often outspoken. When out of balance, they are short-tempered, agitated, jealous, critical, and argumentative. They can become reckless, highly competitive, demanding, and hostile. In any stressful situation, the pitta's typical response is, "What did *you* do wrong?"

As we saw earlier, pittas are focused and competitive. They have a strong desire to win, due to which they can become workaholics and burn out easily. Also, when they meet with resistance, or when things don't go their way, they may become agitated, angry, frustrated, or jealous of others who have accomplished success. This habit leads to gaining more enemies than friends. Pittas need to acknowledge that one cannot attract bees with vinegar, and, in the same way, one cannot build nurturing relationships with a judgmental, critical, and demanding nature. The emotional quotient is an essential skill to succeed in life. There is an expression that says, "To go fast in life, go alone, but to go far, go with a team of like-minded individuals." Hence, pittas must learn to be mindful and observant about their emotions.

Slow down when needed. Celebrate your small accomplishments. Develop people skills and learn to chill. Learn to work with others and appreciate their qualities. A "my way or the highway" mentality does not help anyone. The most important quality a pitta needs to develop is unconditional acceptance and unconditional love toward self and others. While it is important to be nonjudgmental toward self and others, it is essential to show love and compassion toward self before we work on loving and accepting others, because a person who cannot love and accept themselves will not be able to show grace and acceptance toward others.

Balancing Pitta:

The same principles of samanya and vishesha, which we discussed earlier, apply here in balancing an out-of-balance pitta. As we saw earlier, when any dosha is out of balance, Ayurveda recommends the use of the five senses to bring it back into balance.

Balancing by Taste: The best tastes to pacify a pitta are sweet, bitter, and astringent. Minimize foods that are sour, salty, and pungent tastes. To counterbalance the hot nature of the pitta dosha, Ayurveda traditionally recommends foods that are cooling.

Balancing by Touch: To balance pitta, perform deep-tissue massage with cooling oils like coconut oil.

Balancing by Sound: To balance an unbalanced pitta mind, choose soothing sounds like falling rain, waterfalls, sounds of the ocean, soft jazz, flute, and other calming sounds. Choose relaxing music, which can keep you calm.

Balancing by Sight: The out-of-balance pitta mind can be balanced with soft, cool colors, like blues, whites, and greens.

Balancing by Smell: Cooling, soothing, and sweet flowery aromas, such as sandalwood, jasmine, rose, and lavender, can help balance the pitta mind

Pitta types can get very competitive; hence they have to be very careful when they exercise so that they do not overexert themselves or hurt themselves by over-exercising. In Part II of the book, we shall learn more about the types of exercises that are beneficial for pitta-type individuals.

When angry and agitated, pitta types tend to eat their anger. When they cannot let out their anger, they tend to become emotional eaters. As they have a strong digestive fire, they believe that they will be able to digest anything they eat but eating meals when you are emotionally disturbed is not recommended. We read earlier that, at this time, your digestion is weak, and the body cannot digest food properly, producing ama (toxins) from the food you consume. Toxins are gross, heavy, sticky, and they start building up in the tissues and organs. This leads to kapha imbalances in the body.

In another scenario, as pitta types are workaholics, if they take up a highly demanding sales job or management consulting type of job that lacks work-life balance and requires frequent flying and traveling, they may skip meals and not follow a healthy lifestyle habit, that will help them feel grounded. This may cause them to develop anxiety and vata imbalance. The pitta dosha is more prone to become imbalanced, as it is their primary dosha type. One imbalance will lead to an imbalance of the other two doshas as well if the person is not mindful.

In the above-mentioned situations, it is vital that the person is very mindful and addresses the issues from the get-go to avoid worse problems and imbalances. If you are the pitta type, be aware of emotions and anger. Learn healthy coping methods, like journaling or meditation, to control anger instead of becoming an emotional eater. If you need to travel a lot, practice meditation and other grounding techniques to ensure that you do not become anxious or develop vata imbalance.

If you are the pitta type, be aware of emotions and anger. Learn healthy coping methods, like journaling or meditation, to control anger instead of becoming an emotional eater.

Additionally, pittas should avoid hot temperatures, steam rooms, spas, and saunas, too much salty or sour food, fried spicy food, summer heat, and anything which will aggravate or agitate you, like heated arguments.

Passionate Pitta is thy name
Intellect and focus are thy fame
Oh! Without you, who would lead
You are the one that we all need

Earth and water are your best friend
On meditation, you want to depend
Gives you calm and peace
As the poise and grace, you want to increase

Be careful in hot weather
Drink enough water, so you don't wither
Say no to sour and spice
Consume CCF tea and smoothies with lots of ice

While leadership is your strength
Stay calm and cool for a length
Have a heart full of love and patience
So that you can improve all your relations

Pure whites and pastel greens
In between negative thoughts, they will intervene
Slow down and enjoy the journey
Fast and furious makes life murky

Kruti Thakore

Calm Kapha (Endomorph): Structure and Fluidity

Kapha is derived from the water and earth elements. The kapha dosha controls the structure of the body and maintains strength and the physical form in everything, from the bones, muscles, and tendons, right down to the cellular level.

Qualities of Kapha: Qualities of kapha dosha are the same qualities of its elements: earth and water. It is heavy, slow, steady, solid, cold, soft, oily.

Physical Characteristics: Kapha types have a strong build and excellent stamina. They have a large body frame, soft eyes and gaze, smooth and radiant skin, and thick hair. Their joints are well-padded. They have great physical strength, strong willpower, and high endurance. Those who are predominantly kapha sleep soundly and have slow, sluggish digestion. They are the ones who don't like sudden changes, don't like a lot of movement, and don't like to shake things up in their life. This lack of motivation to move and exercise becomes worse when they develop excess kapha. When kapha dosha is out of balance, it manifests in the body as excess weight gain, fluid retention, nasal and chest congestion, allergies, asthma, diabetes, or depression. Just like how too much earth and water combined forms mud, which is sticky, heavy, and gross. In nature, you will observe kapha animals, birds, and plants everywhere. Have you ever seen a swan or goose? Those are examples of kapha birds. Slow, steady, calm. Other examples are elephants, whales, and succulent plants. In any public gathering, you will spot kaphas easily. They patiently listen to the ideas of a vata or are easily led by pittas. At times, you will find them sitting quietly in a corner, hoping no one disturbs them. They naturally are caring and compassionate. When vatas are talking, or pittas are leading, kaphas are listening.

Emotional Characteristics: Calm, collected, content, strong willpower, thoughtful, caring, loving, and compassionate. They have an inherent ability to enjoy life and are comfortable with routine, as it gives them a sense of stability and security.

When in balance, they are strong, willful, loyal, patient, steady, and supportive. When out of balance, they become over-attached to things and people, holding on to jobs and relationships, even if they are no longer nourishing or necessary. Excess kapha in mind will manifest as laziness, sluggishness, resistance to change, withdrawal, indifference, depression, hoarding disorder, lack of motivation, and stubbornness. They can also become shopaholics. In the face of stress, the typical kapha response is, "I don't want to deal with it."

As we saw earlier, kaphas don't like exercise or too much movement, or to get out of their daily routine. It becomes hard to motivate them to exercise or to take up a new challenge for professional growth. Even though they have great endurance and strength, they lack the motivation to get started with exercising or taking calculated risks for their professional growth. Once they start the work, they enjoy it, and they will make sure to complete the task, as they don't give up easily. Hence, kaphas need to identify their "why" or their dream, as it is going to motivate them to start the work. For example, if a kapha type wants to lose weight but is lazy, they should write down their goals, being very specific, and write down how they will feel once they achieve their goals. Keeping an eye on the prize will get them started.

Also, when kaphas meet with resistance, or when things don't go their way, they might become depressed and get drawn to food to seek comfort. As we read earlier, eating when one is emotionally disturbed is not a good idea, and, especially for kapha types, this habit can easily lead to excess kapha, as they have sluggish digestion in the best of circumstances. It is also crucial for them to let go of old habits or toxic relationships that do not serve them well. Instead of withdrawing from any situation and seeking comfort in food, or unnecessary things, they must learn healthy methods to cope with emotions.

Balancing Kapha:

The same principles of samanya and vishesha, which we discussed earlier, apply here in balancing out-of-balance kapha. As we saw earlier, when any dosha is out of balance, Ayurveda recommends the use of the five senses to bring it back into balance.

Balancing by Taste: The best tastes to pacify a kapha are pungent, bitter, and astringent. Minimize foods that are sour, salty, or sweet tastes. To counterbalance the cold and heavy nature of the kapha dosha, Ayurveda traditionally recommends foods that are light and heating.

Balancing by Touch: To balance a kapha, perform a stimulating, vigorous massage with light and warm oils, like sunflower or safflower oils. Also, dry brushing, which is called garshana in Sanskrit, with a soft-bristled body brush can help. One more way to remove excess kapha is by regular use of a steam sauna or dry sauna, as it will promote sweating. Neti pot use is also recommended to remove excess nasal and upper respiratory tract congestion.

Balancing by Sound: To balance an unbalanced kapha mind, choose music that is fast and stimulating so that it can get slow, heavy, and sluggish kapha energy moving. Passionate and fast music, like urban samba, drumbeats, and rock and roll will help.

Balancing by Sight: An out-of-balance kapha mind can be balanced with bold and warm colors like oranges, bright yellows, and red.

Balancing by Smell: Choose stimulating, spicy, and aromatic scents, such as eucalyptus, camphor, clove, juniper, marjoram, and rosemary, to balance an out-of-balance kapha mind.

Exercise and sweat are kapha's best friends, yet kapha types can be very lazy. Hence, they have to be very intentional regarding exercise and movement. We shall go into more detail about exercise and mindful movement in Part II so that you can learn about the benefits of exercise for people with kapha dosha predominance.

Exercise and sweat are kapha's best friends.

When depressed, kapha types tend to eat their depression. As they have a slow digestive fire, this leads to a buildup of toxins which further weakens their digestion. These toxins will build up in the tissues and can make matters worse, leading to excess kapha accumulation, weight gain, and water retention.

Kapha types should avoid cold and heavy meals, frequent eating, cold temperatures, wet and humid weather, ice-cold drinks, too much sweet, salty, or sour food. They should consume warm and light-cooked meals, use lots of spices, favoring spicy, bitter, and astringent tastes.

In ancient Ayurvedic texts, there is a phrase that says "langhanam param aushadham" fasting is the greatest medicine.

In ancient Ayurvedic texts, there is a phrase that says "langhanam param aushadham" fasting is the greatest medicine. In the Ashtanghrudaya, Vagbhatt Rishi lists the benefits of fasting balances all the doshas, removes the accumulated toxins (ama), increases ojas (vitality), boosts the digestive fire, and aids in weight reduction. Fasting might not be for all dosha types, but it benefits people with kapha dosha or those who have kapha imbalance and aggravated kapha dosha. They should favor intermittent fasting and move more.

Calm Kapha is thy name
Loyalty and compassion are thy fame
Oh! Without you, who would care
How we all crave for someone fair

Movement and sweat are your best friend
On exercise, you want to depend
Keeps the sluggishness at bay
Use your strength as you may

As you are prone to weight gain
Your best friends are leafy greens and whole grains
Stand up often and keep moving
On the samba beats, you keep grooving

Shake up your daily routine
Even when you are not at all keen
Spice up your life and meals
Enthusiasm and zest, you shall feel

Bright yellow and brilliant red
Will get you out of your bed
Fast and steady wins the game
Commit to the grind to win the fame

Kruti Thakore

In conclusion, no two people are the same, even if their primary dosha is the same, as they might have a different secondary dosha, so their unique mind-body constitution (prakriti) is different. Also, their vikriti will be different, based on their unique lifestyle. Hence, your prakriti, along with your vikriti, is your unique footprint. We should consider this fact while designing a plan for our optimal well-being.

References:

- *Chopra, D. D., Kshirsagar, D. S., Simon, D. D., Patel, D. S., Porter, D. V., Saint, D. M., Gabriel, R., Stern, E., & Nadarajah, M. (2019, November). The perfect health ayurvedic lifestyle online enrichment program. Session 1–15.*
- *Shilpa, S., & Venkatesha Murthy, C. G. (2011). Understanding personality from Ayurvedic perspective for psychological assessment: A case. Ayu, 32(1), 12–19. https://www.ncbi.nlm.nih.gov/pmc/articles/PMC3215408/*
- *Dey, S., & Pahwa, P. (2014). Prakriti and its associations with metabolism, chronic diseases, and genotypes: Possibilities of newborn screening and a lifetime of personalized prevention. Journal of Ayurveda and integrative medicine, 5(1), 15–24. https://www.ncbi.nlm.nih.gov/pmc/articles/PMC4012357/*
- *Jaiswal, Y. S., & Williams, L. L. (2016). A glimpse of Ayurveda - The forgotten history and principles of Indian traditional medicine. Journal of traditional and complementary medicine, 7(1), 50–53. https://www.ncbi.nlm.nih.gov/pmc/articles/PMC5198827/*
- *Lakhotia S. C. (2014). Translating Ayurveda's Dosha-Prakriti into objective parameters. Journal of Ayurveda and integrative medicine, 5(3), 176. https://www.ncbi.nlm.nih.gov/pmc/articles/PMC4204288/*

CHAPTER 12

Rhythms of Nature and Developing a Daily Routine

T here are five primary rhythms in nature, which govern distinct patterns within the human body. These five rhythms of nature are:

- Circadian rhythms: The 24-hour cycle of night and day
- Seasonal rhythms: The 12-month cycle of the Earth around the sun
- Lunar rhythms: The monthly cycle of the moon around the Earth
- Tidal rhythms: The gravitational influence of the moon on the water
- Celestial rhythms: The rhythms of planetary movement

In this chapter, we will mainly focus on circadian rhythms and seasonal rhythms. Also, we will learn more about how to adjust your daily routine in harmony with circadian rhythms and seasonal rhythms to achieve optimal well-being.

Our bodies and our surrounding environment are interdependent. Our environment is an extension of our physical bodies, and there is a continuous exchange of energy between our bodies and our environment. For example, we inhale oxygen released by the trees surrounding us, and the trees absorb the CO_2 we exhale. We can quote several such examples. Hence, environmental changes have a direct impact on our bodies. Any disruption in our environment will disrupt our mental, emotional, and physical well-being.

These changes in our environment and bodies are called biologic rhythms, which fall into three categories: seasonal, circadian, and ultradian rhythms. Just like living beings, seasons, as well as our days and nights, are divided into vata, pitta, and kapha times. We call circadian rhythms "dinacharya" in Sanskrit, while seasonal rhythms are called "ritucharya."

In Ayurveda, the importance of a consistent daily routine can't be understated. A daily routine sets the tone for our entire day, bringing a sense of calm and well-being. It gives the body, mind, and spirit the chance to ground and cleanse, to start fresh.

It is a great idea to sync our daily routine with circadian rhythms to achieve optimal wellness.

Circadian rhythms are governed by our body's internal clock, and they regulate feelings of sleepiness and wakefulness, as well as body temperature and various hormonal changes, for approximately 24 hours. Our circadian rhythms are aligned with nature's cycle of light and dark, which is why our body is naturally alert and awake when the sun rises and naturally slows down when it gets dark.

Let's look at circadian rhythms and learn to develop dosha-specific daily routines that are in harmony with circadian rhythms.

As we saw in an earlier chapter, vatas do not like routine, but the habit of developing a daily routine will be beneficial for them. At the same time, even though kapha types should bring variety into their day, it is still important for them to have a daily routine while bringing in the variety by changing their exercises or bringing variety into their diet.

In the morning, 6 a.m. to 10 a.m. is kapha time in nature. Everything is slow and sluggish. It is a time when the world is slowly waking up. Kapha types should wake up before 6 a.m. so that they can beat the slow sluggish kapha energy of the morning. Once you wake up, prepare your body for the day. Wash your face with cold or warm water, as per your liking and the weather. For example, pitta types can use cold water, while vata and kapha types should use warm water.

After completing your morning routine, brush your teeth, cleanse the tongue with a tongue cleaner or tongue scraper, and do oil pulling. This will help remove toxins and residue from the tongue and gums. I have observed that, once I started oil pulling, my gums never bleed when I go for dental cleanings. Did you know we have approximately 10,000 taste buds on our tongue? When we keep the tongue clean, we develop a better sense of taste, so we will not require extra salt or sugar on our food to make it taste better.

This is also the best time to do meditation, no matter what your dosha is, as our minds are very quiet early in the morning. Especially if you are vata or pitta type, this will help you calm down and focus on your day. Hence, incorporate meditation into your morning routine.

Then, consume a full glass of warm water with the juice of half a lemon and a teaspoon of organic honey. If you prefer apple cider vinegar or kombucha, you can also incorporate one of those into your morning routine instead of warm water and lemon. This is to awaken our digestive tract, encouraging bowel movement. A healthy bowel movement every morning indicates that our digestive tract is healthy.

A kapha type, or someone with excess kapha, can add one teaspoon of fresh ginger juice, a pinch of salt, and a black pepper powder to their glass of warm water and lemon juice. This will help them ignite the digestive fire.

You can also have a light breakfast in the morning if you wish. Pitta types should never skip breakfast because they get angry when hungry, while kapha types can do without breakfast, or just with a light breakfast, like a fruit or a boiled egg, for example. The key is to be mindful and listen to your body. Only eat if you are hungry.

For people who feel very sluggish in the morning, I recommend exercising before 10 a.m. If you have a busy schedule, then at least go for a quick 30-minute walk, jog, or bike ride, or do quick sun salutations and pranayama, of course, depending on your health situation and the capacity of your body. Use common sense and discernment. This will energize your body and help you remove the sluggishness.

For people who feel very sluggish in the morning, I recommend exercising before 10 a.m.

Also, if your schedule and your skin condition permits, you can allocate more time in the morning toward self-care and do dry brushing or abhyanga (oil massage). Dry brushing helps remove dead skin cells, stimulates the lymphatic system, exfoliates the skin, helps the body get rid of toxins, increases circulation and energy, and helps break down cellulite. Abhyanga helps to improve circulation, soothes skin, strengthens tissues, and lubricates joints. Again, if you have sensitive skin or any skin disease, consult your doctor before performing dry brushing or abhyanga. Showering or taking a bath is one more important morning routine that follows abhyanga or dry brushing, as it will make you feel alert and energize you. People who have allergies or sinus congestion can incorporate the use of neti pot and nasya therapy in their morning routine.

10 a.m. to 2 p.m. is pitta time. This is the time when our digestive fire is at its peak. This is when we can have our lunch. I recommend that lunch should be the heaviest meal of the day, but, at the same time, it should be nourishing and balanced so that you don't feel sluggish after lunch. Also, follow the simple guidelines and try to incorporate all six tastes in your meals. The six tastes are sweet, salty, sour, bitter, pungent, and astringent. At the same time, have a dosha-specific diet. For example, kapha types should reduce sweet, salty, and sour tastes in their meals and increase bitter, pungent, and astringent tastes. Hence, it is crucial to learn about your dosha or prakriti, as well as vikriti, so that you can follow dosha-specific guidelines to achieve optimal well-being.

2 p.m. to 6 p.m. is vata time. If you had a nourishing lunch, the food would fuel your creativity and improve your focus. This is the best time for creativity. If you had a heavy, dull meal full of carbs and fat, you might feel sluggish.

6 p.m. to 10 p.m. is kapha time. This is the time to wind down. If you observe nature, everything is winding down. This is the time when the digestive fire is slow. Hence, dinner should be light and eaten, at the latest, by 7 p.m. Also, do not exercise or use caffeine after 6 p.m., or your sleep will be disturbed. Try to wind down so that you can hit the bed by 10 p.m.

10 p.m. to 2 a.m. is pitta time. This is the time when our body repairs and rejuvenates. Pitta, or digestion, is not as strong as it is during the pitta time during the day. During this time, your body will digest the meal you had at dinner, but as the body is asleep, the energy is spent in maintaining body heat and keeping you warm, as well as in building and repairing tissues. The body metabolizes whatever it takes in through our five senses, including food and experiences. It removes toxins and repairs itself. We recommend going to bed by 10

p.m. so that you can help your body repair itself. I also recommend meditation before bedtime instead of watching movies or news. Meditation will calm you down, quiet your mind, and improve the quality of your sleep.

2 a.m. to 6 a.m. is, again, vata time. During this time, the air and space elements are dominant in nature, as well as in our minds and bodies. During this time, as vata dominates the environment and our nervous system, our mind becomes very active. You will more likely have a busy or agitated mind due to vata, which can quickly become overactive or anxious, making falling asleep very difficult. Hence, if you wake up during this time, it becomes difficult to fall asleep again.

While circadian rhythm is our body's natural internal process, which regulates our internal clock and repeats every 24 hours, we also need to learn how to assist our bodies to cope with seasonal rhythms. There are six seasons in general, and many countries, experience all six of them. But here in the United States, we experience four main seasons: spring, summer, autumn, and winter. When we transition from one season to another, we experience several changes, from a change in the temperature and humidity to daylight savings time. These changes put our bodies into mild shock and cause several disruptions in our bodies. We experience several changes at a cellular level, and, most importantly, our bodies also undergo hormonal changes. Studies have shown that our bodies also must adjust when nature is adjusting to the seasonal changes. Winter blues are as real as spring allergies. Hence, we must facilitate our bodies to go through these changes smoothly so that we can have optimal health.

Studies have shown that our bodies also must adjust when nature is adjusting to the seasonal changes. Winter blues are as real as spring allergies.

Late Autumn and Winter – Vata Time
Spring and Early Summer – Kapha Time
Summer and Early Autumn – Pitta Time

During late autumn and winter, the weather is cold and dry. Days become shorter, and nights are longer. Sunsets are early, and it is dark before 5 p.m. This is the vata season, as per Ayurveda. People may experience a vata imbalance. Depending on their dosha type, some people experience winter blues or mild depression, or anxiety. Our hair and skin become dry. Our nasal passages become irritated due to dryness. Our ability to focus reduces. This is the time to include neti pot and nasya therapy in your daily routine, even if you usually do not include them. Consume warm, easily digestible meals. Feel free to include healthy fats in your diet.

During late winter, spring, and early summer, the weather has started to warm up. There is moisture in the air, and it rains often. That's why it is said, "April showers bring May flowers." This is kapha season. Many people experience sluggishness, and mucus may build up in their nasal passages and sinuses. This is allergy and flu season for many. Continue the practice of using the neti pot to remove mucus and prevent sinus infections. Consume warm and light meals.

During summer through early autumn, the weather is scorching and dry. At times, we experience heat waves. Rivers and water bodies are drying up. This is the pitta season. People may become dehydrated and tired quickly. People with sensitive skin may get heat rashes. Hunger is reduced, as well as energy levels. Some people get angry and agitated often.

Early autumn and early spring are also considered transitional seasons. In early autumn, we are transitioning from hot and dry summer months, the pitta season, to cold and dry autumn, the vata season. In early spring, we are transitioning from cold and dry winter, vata season, to warm and damp spring, kapha season. During these times, our immunity is reduced, as our bodies are going through internal changes and, hence, people are prone to flu, cold, cough, allergies, mucous buildup, sinus infections, etc. Be extra careful during seasons that match your unique mind-body constitution/ dosha. For example, pitta-type people should be cautious in summer, while kapha-type people should be cautious in late winter and spring.

While you already learned about how to set a healthy daily routine, here are a few tips on how to reset the metabolism, which is affected during all these seasonal changes:

- Early autumn and early spring are the perfect times to do a gentle detox so that you can reset your metabolism. You can use herbs like Triphala for a gentle detox. Also, starting your day with the juice of half a lemon in warm water helps detox your system.
- As I mentioned earlier, Ayurveda says "langhanam param aushadham," which means "fasting is the best medicine." Intermittent fasting, liquid diet, or juice detox will help to remove toxins and ignite the digestive fire. Khichdi is an ideal food for detox.
- Always wear comfortable clothing. Warm clothes when it is cold and light cotton when it is warm.
- Incorporate physical activity and exercise into your daily routine.
- Meditate and practice mindful eating.
- Your lunch should be the heartiest meal, and dinner should always be light. Warm soups as dinner in cold months, and refreshing salads as dinner in hot months, can be ideal. Also, don't consume meals at least four hours before bedtime, and don't overeat.

- Consume warm, freshly cooked meals cooked with dosha-specific spices, like ginger, cloves, peppers, garlic, onions, turmeric, fennel, oregano, thyme, etc., during autumn and winter months. Sip on warm liquids, like herbal teas and warm water, throughout the day. This will help you to remove mucus and ignite your digestive fire. Consume seasonal vegetables and fruits.

- Consume warm and light meals that are easy to digest during transitional seasons and kapha season. Include spices that aid your digestion, as, during this period, digestion is very sluggish.

- Consume light, refreshing meals during the hot season. Cucumbers, watermelon, yogurt, dill, fennel, mint, coconut, melons, green leafy vegetables cooked with gentle spices, etc., are ideal for these months. Sip on cold liquids and cold herbal teas to stay hydrated. You don't have to use ice if your dosha is kapha or vata, but instead of consuming warm fluids, you can drink fluids at room temperature. If your dosha is pitta, feel free to add some ice cubes to the water or tea you consume. The bottom line is to listen to your body and stay hydrated.

- Develop a regular practice of nasyam and use of the neti pot, especially during kapha seasons or if your primary dosha is kapha.

- Incorporating the practices of abhyanga (massage with warm oil) and dry brushing also are beneficial. As mentioned in the previous chapter, you can use the oil as per your dosha type.

- Get a good night's sleep of at least eight hours and maintain a daily sleep routine. Try to avoid late nights and irregular sleep times. Follow circadian rhythms.

In addition to nurturing your body with the proper diet, it is essential to nurture your mind and spirit for emotional well-being.

References:

- *Chopra, D. D., Kshirsagar, D. S., Simon, D. D., Patel, D. S., Porter, D. V., Saint, D. M., Gabriel, R., Stern, E., & Nadarajah, M. (2019, November). The perfect health ayurvedic lifestyle online enrichment program. Session 1–15.*
- *U.S. Department of Health and Human Services. (n.d.). Circadian rhythms. National Institute of General Medical Sciences. Retrieved December 26, 2021, from https://www.nigms.nih.gov/education/fact-sheets/Pages/circadian-rhythms.aspx*
- *Thakkar, J., Chaudhari, S., & Sarkar, P. K. (2011). Ritucharya: Answer to the lifestyle disorders. Ayu, 32(4), 466–471. https://www.ncbi.nlm.nih.gov/pmc/articles/PMC3361919/*

CHAPTER 13

Panchakarma

_₭₭₭_

Panchakarma is the Ayurvedic method of detoxification and rejuvenation. Pancha in Sanskrit means "five," and karma means "action," so panchakarma means "five actions" to detoxify and rejuvenate. Panchakarma practice should only be done by, or under the supervision of, an Ayurvedic practitioner or Ayurvedic doctor. Panchakarma helps restore digestive fire, eliminate toxins, and restore the balance of all three doshas. Normally it is performed from five days to a maximum of 21 days, depending on the type of problems the patient or person receiving the treatment is facing.

Research has shown that people who undergo panchakarma therapy have a significant decrease in chronic inflammation and a huge improvement in their physical, emotional, and mental well-being. As I mentioned, panchakarma is a combination of five procedures, which focus on purification and removing deep-rooted imbalances in the body through vamana (emesis), virechana (purgation), nirooha vasti (decoction enema), nasya (instillation of medicine through the nostrils), and anuvasanavasti (oil enema).

You might ask, Are detoxification and rejuvenation necessary?

We live in a hectic, stressful, and toxic world. Due to the fast lifestyle and chemicals, from inorganic farming practices to cleaning products in our environment, the water and air quality are deteriorating, and so is the quality of our life. Due to this, our minds and bodies accumulate toxins, which results in imbalances in our minds and bodies as well as deterioration of our health. This opens the door for chronic inflammation, resulting in degenerative and lifestyle-related diseases, ultimately damaging an individual's health and wellness.

Panchakarma helps to reverse these effects and brings harmony to your mind and body. It restores your natural state of health and wellness by eliminating toxins from your body and improving bodily functions. The focus is on the prevention of disease instead of cure by removing the toxins and preventing further production of toxins by changing one's lifestyle and diet. Once the panchakarma is completed, over several days, Ayurveda strongly recommends changing lifestyle habits, diet, and incorporating exercise into your daily routine so you can stop further damage. It is not a quick fix, but it is the beginning of lifestyle change. If you are not committed to changing your lifestyle, you will find yourself in the same situation a couple of years down the road.

> *The focus is on the prevention of disease instead of cure by removing the toxins and preventing further production of toxins by changing one's lifestyle and diet.*

Traditional Panchakarma vs. Modern Panchakarma

Ayurvedic practices have been around for more than 5000 years, and panchakarma has evolved throughout those years.

In ancient times, panchakarma therapy included five actions as mentioned below:

1. Basti: Herbal oil enema
2. Nasya: Nasal irrigation
3. Vamana: Therapeutic vomiting
4. Virechana: Purgation
5. Raktamokshana: Bloodletting for purification of blood

These treatments have been modified in current times, and nowadays, a panchakarma program includes the following:

1. Abhyanga (herbal oil deep-tissue massage), garshana (dry brushing), and udvartanam (deep-tissue massage using dry herbal powder)
2. Swedna: Steam bath
3. Elimination of toxins through one or more of several methods, like herbal oil enema, vamana (therapeutic vomiting), virechana (purgation), senna (gentle laxatives), anuvasanavasti (oil enema).
4. Nasya: Nasal irrigation
5. Specialized diet and herbal supplements

In addition to these five basic steps, your Ayurvedic doctor or practitioner may incorporate several other treatments, like shirodhara (to promote relaxation), katibasti (treatment for lumbar and back support), janu basti (treatment for knee joints), nabhi basti (to promote digestion), netra basti (treatment for vision health), etc., depending on your unique needs.

In Ayurveda, it is firmly believed that, as everyone is unique, so are their needs, and there is no one-size-fits-all approach. Hence, panchakarma must be performed under the supervision of an Ayurvedic doctor or certified Ayurvedic practitioner. I, personally, was fortunate to experience panchakarma therapy, which healed me from excess kapha imbalance and severe allergies. For me, the whole experience was a powerful journey into healing and rejuvenation.

Steps Before Panchakarma

Before the panchakarma therapy, your Ayurvedic practitioner will prepare your body with some of the above-mentioned methods, like abhyanga and swedna, so that it will let go of the toxins. In abhyanga, using warm herbal oil, the practitioner will perform the deep-tissue massage that

Panchakarma must be performed under the supervision of an Ayurvedic doctor or certified Ayurvedic practitioner.

facilitates tissues, organs, and cells to release toxins and move them toward the gastrointestinal tract. This also removes stress, nourishes the nervous system, and makes the tissues soft and supple.

After abhyanga, sweating is induced through a steam sauna. This process is called swedna. An herbal concoction may be added to the steam to further loosen the toxins. Through abhyanga and swedna, the toxins are released into the gastrointestinal tract and then, using one method, or a combination of the methods mentioned above, the toxins are eliminated from the GI tract. A particular panchakarma method is then given as per the individual's constitution and disorder, prakriti, and vikriti. During the complete treatment, you might also be prescribed diet restrictions and herbal supplements.

Benefits:

- Eliminates toxins from your body and mind.
- Facilitates healing of lifestyle-related illnesses.
- Restores, repairs, relaxes, and rejuvenates at a cellular level

- Restores balance to your dosha (mind-body constitution) to improve overall health and well-being.
- Strengthens your immune system.
- Slows down the aging process by reversing the adverse effects of stress on your body and mind.
- Enhances the sense of well-being.
- Improves flexibility, resilience, strength, energy, vitality, and mental clarity.

As the panchakarma therapy is not easily accessible in all the parts of the world, and it can also be expensive, in the next chapter we will review how you can incorporate some of the practices into your daily routine, along with eating a wholesome, life-supporting diet and incorporating exercise to promote self-care.

References:

- *Chopra, D. D., Kshirsagar, D. S., Simon, D. D., Patel, D. S., Porter, D. V., Saint, D. M., Gabriel, R., Stern, E., & Nadarajah, M. (2019, November). The perfect health ayurvedic lifestyle online enrichment program. Session 1–15.*
- *Conboy, L., Edshteyn, I., & Garivaltis, H. (2009). Ayurveda and Panchakarma: measuring the effects of a holistic health intervention. The Scientific World Journal, 9, 272–280. https://www.ncbi.nlm.nih.gov/pmc/articles/mid/NIHMS116241/*
- *Rawal, M., Chudasma, K. M., Vyas, R. V., & Parmar, B. P. (2010). Effect of Vasantic Vaman and other Panchakarma procedures on disorders of various systems. Ayu, 31(3), 319–324. https://www.ncbi.nlm.nih.gov/pmc/articles/PMC3221065/*

CHAPTER 14

Incorporating Self-care into Daily Routine: Neti pot, Nasya, Oil Pulling, Swedna, Abhyanga, Dry Brushing, and Eye Exercises

※≪←

We saw in our earlier chapter that, to achieve physical and emotional well-being, it is essential to maintain a daily routine that is in harmony with circadian and seasonal rhythms. In this chapter, we shall discuss the benefits of several self-care techniques, like using a neti pot, nasya, oil pulling, swedna, abhyanga, dry brushing, etc., which can be incorporated into your daily routine to enhance the quality of your health and life.

What is a neti pot and what are the benefits of using one?

On one spring afternoon in 2018, I started experiencing severe headaches and postnasal drip. I could not figure out the reason, so I visited my doctor, and they thought I might have caught a sinus infection or cold virus from swimming. I was recommended to stop swimming for a week or two and take antibiotics. I felt a bit better, but then the symptoms became more severe. I developed severe postnasal drip, was constantly coughing, and could not sleep. Finally, I visited a specialist, and, after allergy tests, I found out that I had developed severe allergies to almost 16 different things, including dust mites, grass, and tree pollen. I was put on allergy medication, which caused severe gastric problems and hyperacidity, so I tried immunotherapy for almost six months, but I did not experience any relief.

At that point, I was introduced to a course from The Chopra Center in Perfect Health Ayurvedic Lifestyle. My inner instincts nudged me to pursue this certification course, and I started learning about the Ayurvedic lifestyle. I started implementing what I learned into my daily routine, and within a few weeks, I saw a difference. Along with making changes in my daily routine, I also visited an Ayurvedic doctor and started panchakarma treatment. With the help of a change in my diet, daily routine, and treatment, my allergies are 95 percent cured. Since then, I have incorporated the neti pot in my daily morning routine and have experienced tremendous benefits.

If you want to incorporate the use of a neti pot into your daily routine, you can search for instructions videos on YouTube to learn the technique. A neti pot is a very popular home-based remedy for nasal congestion. It is a personal hygiene practice for nasal irrigation and has several benefits. One can purchase a neti pot online or from a local pharmacy.

Benefits of Using a Neti Pot:

- Clears the nostrils to facilitate easy breathing
- Removes excess mucus
- Clears sinuses, releases sinus and nasal congestion
- Eases sinus headaches
- Soothes dry nasal passages
- Reduces the need for antiallergy medicines
- Reduces pollen or allergens in nasal passages
- Relieves nasal dryness
- Reduces cold and flu symptoms
- Alleviates sinus headaches
- Improves sense of smell and taste
- Prevents upper respiratory infections and cold
- Reduces snoring

Here are some tips on how to use a neti pot (despite the helpfulness of the following tips, I recommend watching instruction videos on YouTube before using it):

- I prefer a ceramic neti pot, but you can buy a good quality ceramic, glass, or metal neti pot from a local pharmacy or the internet.
- You will also need neti salt.
- A typical neti pot looks like Aladdin's magic lamp and holds about one cup of water, to which you will add approximately one teaspoon of neti salt. When you buy neti salt, you will get a measuring spoon with it. Just use that measuring spoon.
- Use distilled, sterile, or filtered water. The water temperature should be lukewarm. Dip your finger in the water to feel the temperature. Water temperature should not be too cold or too

hot. I warm the water on the stove. Wash your hands before dipping your finger in the water.

- Add neti salt to the lukewarm water and fill the neti pot with the warm saltwater. To avoid stinging, use non-iodized salt and make sure it is completely dissolved in the water.

- Place the spout of the neti pot in one nostril and gently pour in the warm salt water while breathing with the mouth. Your head should be positioned at about a 45-degree angle, so the water runs out the other nostril. Repeat the process on the other nostril. Be sure to clean your neti pot after each use.

Sometimes we feel that, after using the neti pot, there is still some water in the nasal passages, and this water drips when we look down. Nothing to worry about. This is natural. I use the neti pot in the morning before consuming anything, and immediately after using the neti pot, I do Kapalbhati pranayama, which helps me remove excess water from the nasal passages. You can watch YouTube videos to learn Kapalbhati pranayama.

Tip: Use a neti pot before taking a plane flight to moisten your breathing passages.

For severe allergies and sinus congestion, after using the neti pot, you can inhale steam vapors and perform nasya.

Use a neti pot before taking a plane flight to moisten your breathing passages.

Nasya Therapy

As I mentioned earlier, the neti pot and panchakarma therapy healed my severe allergies. In traditional Ayurvedic practice, nasya is a part of panchakarma treatment for body cleansing used in Ayurvedic medicine. Nasya uses the route of the nasal cavity to administer ayurvedic herbs into our upper respiratory tract. Nasya

Therapy, during panchakarma therapy, must be only performed by an Ayurvedic doctor in their clinic, so how can one reap the benefits of nasya at home?

Before we get into the details, here are a few benefits of Nasya Kriya, or nasya therapy:

- Nasya lubricates the nasal membrane, especially after using a neti pot, as nasya oil nourishes and lubricates freshly cleaned nasal passages.

- During winters, when heaters run in our homes, especially in the northern hemisphere, our nose sometimes bleeds as it dries up. The neti pot and nasya therapy can help moisturize our nasal passages and prevent bleeding from the nose.

- Nasya treatment can be helpful with headaches, migraines, sinus congestion, allergies, nose bleeds, dry nasal passages, and insomnia.

- I recommend inhaling steam after using a neti pot and before you perform nasya therapy. The main benefit of inhaling moist, warm steam is that it can ease irritation and reduce the swelling of the blood vessels in the nasal passages. It can also loosen up the mucus in your sinuses, so you can remove it from the nose more easily and help relieve nasal congestion and headaches.

- Pacifies vata dosha.

Nasya treatment can be helpful with headaches, migraines, sinus congestion, allergies, nose bleeds, dry nasal passages, and insomnia.

Method:

- Cleanse nasal passage with a neti pot.
- Inhale steam for 10 to 15 minutes by carefully pouring boiling water in a large pot, draping a towel around your head, shutting your eyes, and lowering your face until you are approximately a foot away from the hot water. Inhale slowly and deeply. Be very careful not to make direct contact with the hot water. If you prefer an easier method, use a facial steamer. You can also add camphor oil or eucalyptus oil to the steamer. Inhaling steam will clear your nasal passages and loosen the mucus.
- Choose organic sesame/almond/olive oil. You can buy nasya oil from Amazon or any other authentic website. Sesame oil is best for nasya, as it is warm, grounding, and calming. Also, it is highly nourishing and moisturizing. It can bring deep relief to dry, irritated, or congested nasal passages when performed after using a neti pot and after inhaling steam.
- Place a drop of the oil on your clean pinky and apply it gently inside your nostril. Then gently inhale so that the oil penetrates the nasal membranes. Repeat on another side. If you are comfortable, you can always use a dropper instead of your finger to put two to three drops of oil in your nose. If you are using a dropper, you will need to lie down comfortably or sit down in a reclining chair and tilt your head backward. Hold your breath, keep the dropper about one-half inch above your nose, add two to three drops in each nasal passage and inhale. Stay in this position for five to ten minutes and inhale before you get up.
- If needed, you can gently tap or massage your nose so that the oil spreads evenly.
- Recommended during cold weather or spring when the air is filled with pollen and dust.

- Nasya should not be administered immediately after a bath, after a meal, during pregnancy, or to those who have undergone nasal surgery. It is not advised for children under seven years or people over eighty years.
- If you have any serious medical condition, please consult your doctor before performing nasya therapy. If you experience discomfort while using the neti pot, inhaling steam, or performing nasya therapy, do not continue, and consult your doctor.

Oil Pulling

Oil pulling is done in the morning after you wake up. It is an alternative medical practice in which one takes an organic, edible oil, usually sesame or coconut oil, and swish it around in the mouth for 20 minutes or so, like a mouth wash, then spits it out. Start with 10 minutes, and then slowly increase. It might feel weird initially, but with practice you will get used to it. You don't have to brush your teeth and clean your tongue with a tongue scraper before oil pulling, but make sure to do so after oil pulling.

Oil pulling helps remove toxins from your mouth, tongue, and gums. It has several benefits, like improving your oral health and whitening your teeth, reducing the harmful bacteria in your mouth, cleansing your taste buds by removing toxins, so the food you eat will taste better, thus helping you avoid adding excess salt or other seasonings to your food. It can also improve the health of your gums, reduce your risk of cavities, and eliminate bad breath. Since I started oil pulling, I have seen that my gums do not bleed when I go for regular dental cleanings. It can also improve your overall health and wellness by drawing toxins out of the body.

Oil pulling helps remove toxins from your mouth, tongue, and gums.

Swedna

Swedna is a Sanskrit word derived from sweda, which means "sweat or perspiration." Swedna means "a method to induce sweating and perspiration." As we saw earlier, sweat is the enemy of fat, and our body also removes toxins through perspiration. Swedna is an Ayurvedic therapy where toxins are removed through perspiration, using herbal steam, and it is an essential part of panchakarma practice. Our sweat glands help us remove toxins through the act of sweating. There are thousands of sweat glands located on our skin, and, when stimulated, they can help in mobilizing the toxins in the inner layers of the skin and muscles so that we can get rid of them.

Even though swedna is performed under the supervision of the Ayurvedic practitioner, one can reap the benefits of swedna at home by using a steam sauna or dry sauna. There are several inexpensive options available in the market. Just do proper research and due diligence before purchasing one. I, personally, prefer a steam sauna over a dry or infrared sauna because my skin is dry, and it gets irritated with dry heat from the sauna. Mindfulness is the key here, so listen to your body's needs. Also, keep the duration under 45 minutes. If you are using a sauna at a gym or home, consume at least one to two glasses of warm water during the winter and cold water during warmer weather before and after using the sauna.

There are thousands of sweat glands located on our skin, and, when stimulated, they can help in mobilizing the toxins in the inner layers of the skin and muscles so that we can get rid of them.

Benefits of Swedna

When the body gets heated, there is an increase in blood flow, which facilitates the removal of toxins, as well as a continuous supply of nutrients at a deep cellular level. Also, heat transforms toxins into a simple form for easy removal. Thus, swedna promotes detoxification and removes deep-rooted ama or toxins.

- Relieves muscular tension.
- Restores flexibility
- Clears energy passages.
- Helps with muscular inflammation, hypertension, blood pressure, and circulation.
- Improves blood flow in the skin and tissues, resulting in well-nourished skin. Thus, it softens skin and improves the luster of skin.
- Heat increases metabolic rate and facilitates the burning of fats.
- Improves joint mobility.
- Relieves aches and pains.
- Reduces stress and fatigue.
- Activates circulation and improves varicose veins.
- Improves metabolism and appetite.
- Improves kidney function and aids digestion.
- Helps to control arthritic problems.

If you feel any kind of discomfort, do not continue the practice. Most importantly, stay hydrated, and drink a glass of warm water before and after using a sauna. It is not recommended for pregnant women or someone who suffers from dizziness, vertigo, and other disorders.

Abhyanga

The Ayurvedic abhyanga, or oil massage, is one of the most important aspects of the daily routine. Like swedna, abhyanga is also a crucial part of panchakarma practice. Here we shall discuss the benefits of abhyanga and how you can perform it at home. Abhyanga promotes healing through touch, as the sense of touch promotes emotional and psychological healing. Abhyanga has healing benefits to the endocrine system and nervous system. Abhyanga benefits include improving circulation; nourishing tissues, improving skin health, moisture, and luster; aiding in detoxification, improving immunity, lubricating joints and tissues, and improving sleep. It also promotes lymphatic drainage and reduces muscle stiffness.

> *Abhyanga benefits include improving circulation; nourishing tissues, improving skin health, moisture, and luster; aiding in detoxification, improving immunity, lubricating joints and tissues, and improving sleep.*

Instructions for a Performing Abhyanga

- Select dosha-appropriate oil. People who have out-of-balance vata dosha, or who have vata dosha as their dominant dosha, should use heavy, warm oils, like sesame or almond. A light touch is recommended for using either. People with excess pitta dosha, or with pitta dosha predominance, will benefit from deep-tissue massages with cooling oils, such as coconut, sunflower, or olive. People with kapha dosha predominance, or with excess kapha, will benefit from a stimulating, vigorous massage with lighter oils, such as safflower or sunflower, or warmer oils like mustard or almond.

- Gently heat a small quantity of oil. The best place to perform your massage is your bathroom. You might want to cover the floor with a large towel. While massaging your body, show love and respect for your body. Your state of mind is equally as important as the technique. A loving touch will promote healing and relaxation.

- Start with the scalp by pouring a tablespoon of warm oil onto your scalp and massaging it gently, in circular motions, with your fingertips, as if you were shampooing your hair.

- Next, with light, gentle strokes, apply the oil to your forehead, cheeks, and chin, in circular and upward motions. Massage the backs of your ears and temples, and then apply a little more oil to your hands and massage the front and back of your neck.

- Then, massage your arms, using a circular motion at the shoulders and elbows and long, back-and-forth motions on the upper arms and forearms. Massage using large, gentle, circular motions on your chest, stomach, and lower abdomen, while using a straight up-and-down motion over the breastbone. Apply oil in your palms and gently massage your back and spine the best you can.

- Next, vigorously massage your legs, just like you did your arms, using circular motions at the ankles and knees, with back-and-forth motions on the long parts. With the remaining bit of oil, vigorously massage your feet. Pay extra attention to your toes. Sit quietly for a few moments to let the oil soak into your body.

- You must wait for 20 to 25 minutes after you finish your massage before you take a shower or bath. After that, rinse your body with warm water and mild soap, which will help you maintain a light film of oil.

Mini Massage

Sometimes, you might not have time to do a full-body massage; in that case, you can perform a mini massage. At least something is better than nothing. Similarly, a short one is still much better than none. When you lack time to perform a full-body massage, focus on the head and feet, as they are the most important parts of the body. The mini massage requires only about two tablespoons of oil.

- Rub one tablespoon of warm oil into your scalp, forehead, and temples, and then lightly rub your ears. Spend a few moments massaging the back and front of your neck.
- With the second tablespoon of oil, massage both feet using the flats of your hands, and then rub your toes with your fingertips. Lastly, vigorously massage the soles of your feet with brisk back-and-forth motions of the palms.

Dry Brushing

Ayurvedic dry brushing, or garshana, is a technique done with raw silk or linen gloves or a brush with coarse natural-fiber bristles brushed over the skin. Dry brushing helps you remove dead skin, as brushing the skin when it is dry exfoliates it and increases blood circulation. It opens up the clogged pores and aids detoxification, as it helps to drain lymphatic fluids. Garshana is stimulating and is very helpful in balancing excess kapha. Choose a brush with a long handle so that you can easily reach your back.

Dry brushing helps you remove dead skin, as brushing the skin when it is dry exfoliates it and increases blood circulation.

Tips on Performing Dry Brushing

As mentioned above, use a natural-fiber brush with a long handle so that you can reach all the areas of your body.

- Using gloves or a brush, massage vigorously to stimulate the skin and lymph nodes.
- Brush in broad circular strokes.
- If you are new to dry brushing, apply gentle pressure initially until you get used to dry brushing.
- Start with your feet and move up, as strokes should always be toward the heart.
- Brush your arms, trunk, and then brush your armpits in an upward motion.
- Take a shower to remove the dry skin. If you want, you can do abhyanga with dosha-specific oil before showering.
- If you prefer not to do abhyanga after dry brushing, you can immediately take your shower. After the shower, pat dry and moisturize your skin with natural oil, like olive oil, almond oil, or coconut oil.

Avoid sensitive areas, and any place where the skin is broken. Do not dry brush your face. Dry brushing might not work if you have sensitive skin, or very dry skin, so be very mindful and listen to your body. In the case of sensitive or dry skin, you can use a gentle sugar scrub or body scrub while enjoying a bubble bath to remove dead skin, if you don't have any skin disease.

Also, never perform dry brushing or abhyanga without checking with your doctor if you have any skin diseases, injuries, irritation, inflammation, sores, scrapes, cuts, lesions, burned skin, or skin cancer. If the brush bristles are very harsh or uncomfortable, you can also try a dry towel or washcloth.

Eye Exercises and Triphala Wash

Along with taking good care of our bodies with the right nutrition and exercise, we also must take good care of our eyes. Nowadays, most of us spend our time in front of a computer or on a smartphone, which strains our eyes. Some people even need prescription eyeglasses at a young age. Over and above that, people frequently experience dry eyes, irritated and itchy eyes, due to lack of sleep, stress, overexposure to electronic devices, and unhealthy lifestyle habits, like reading in dim light or dark. All these habits strain the eyes, so it is essential to take care of our eyes.

Here are some simple exercises for our vision health:

Palming: This is an excellent way to reduce stress on your eyes and relax them. Sit comfortably. Rub your palms together until they are warm. Close your eyes, gently cup your palms, and put them over your eyes. Breathe deeply and repeat it four to five times. Just be gentle and don't put pressure on your eyes while doing this exercise.

Eye Rotations: This is an excellent exercise for your eye muscles. Start by standing or sitting erect. Cover your right eye with your right hand. Take a pencil or pen in your left hand, or clench your fingers and with an erect thumb, and point either the pencil or your thumb directly in front of the nose while keeping your elbow straight. Look at the object (pencil/pen/thumb) with your left eye. Now, move the object up and down, following the object with your left eye, without moving your face or neck. Do this a couple of times, and then move the object left to right, and, similarly, follow the object without moving your head or neck. Finally, rotate the object clockwise and counterclockwise, continuing to follow it as it rotates. Perform this exercise for two to three minutes, and then repeat it with the right eye.

Washing eyes with room temperature water: This is an excellent exercise when you've been working on the computer or watching TV or reading for a couple of hours. It can relax and refresh your eyes. It may also reduce dry-eye syndrome and irritation. Buy a glass eyewash cup. Rinse it thoroughly before every use. Fill it up with sterile room temperature water and wash your eyes by gently tilting your head forward and applying the cup to one eye while preventing the liquid from escaping. Blink your eye a couple of times in the cup. Discard the water. Wash the cup and repeat for another eye.

Triphala eyewash: Repeat the above-mentioned exercise, but instead of using sterile water, you can also prepare a Triphala eyewash and wash your eyes with it. Triphala is an Ayurvedic herb used for its detoxifying and healing properties. Just make sure to buy the organic Triphala powder. Soak one teaspoon powdered Triphala in one cup of sterile water overnight. In the morning, strain the water with a coffee filter to remove any particles, and use that water instead of plain sterile water to wash the eyes. Follow instructions as mentioned above for washing the eyes.

References:

- *Chopra, D. D., Kshirsagar, D. S., Simon, D. D., Patel, D. S., Porter, D. V., Saint, D. M., Gabriel, R., Stern, E., & Nadarajah, M. (2019, November). The perfect health ayurvedic lifestyle online enrichment program. Session 1–15.*
- *Rabago, D., & Zgierska, A. (2009). Saline nasal irrigation for upper respiratory conditions. American family physician, 80(10), 1117–1119. https://www.ncbi.nlm.nih.gov/pmc/articles/PMC2778074/*
- *Shanbhag V. K. (2016). Oil pulling for maintaining oral hygiene - A review. Journal of traditional and complementary medicine, 7(1), 106–109. https://www.ncbi.nlm.nih.gov/pmc/articles/PMC5198813/*

CHAPTER 15

The Consequences of Tobacco, Alcohol, and Drug Addiction

⧁⧁⧁

Tobacco use is a top preventable cause of death. Studies have found that tobacco users are more likely to succumb to alcohol and drug addiction, and people who consume alcohol are more likely to get addicted to smoking and drugs. In short, it is a vicious cycle, with one addiction making people more prone to several others.

As per the survey and research conducted by The National Institute on Alcohol Abuse and Alcoholism (NIAAA) in 2001–2002, approximately 46 million adults used both alcohol and tobacco, and approximately 6.2 million adults reported both Alcohol use disorders (AUD) and nicotine dependence. Codependence on smoking and alcohol puts people at high risk for tobacco-related complications, including multiple cancers, lung disease, and heart disease (e.g., cardiovascular disease). Even though the effects associated with

Codependence on smoking and alcohol puts people at high risk for tobacco-related complications, including multiple cancers, lung disease, and heart disease (e.g., cardiovascular disease).

substance misuse depend on several factors, like the types of substances, how much, how often, and how they are taken, along with several other factors, some of the adverse effects are:

Direct consequences: Alcohol and drugs affect heart rate and regulation of body temperature, can cause psychotic episodes, the possibility of overdose, and death. Research has shown that more people die from alcohol and drug overdoses each year than in automobile accidents. Over and above alcohol and drug abuse, in 2014, nearly 30,000 people died due to drug overdose and prescription opioids. In addition to that, approximately 20,000 people died due to unintentional overdose of alcohol, cocaine, or non-opioid prescription drugs. Substance misuse during pregnancy can result in long-lasting health effects for the baby, and opioid abuse leads to opioid dependency in the newborn. Smoking and tobacco use leads to disease and disability. It harms almost every organ in the body. Tobacco use is linked with the development of chronic obstructive pulmonary disease (COPD), Berger's disease, certain types of cancer, heart disease, stroke, asthma, gum disease, and tooth loss. Smoking may increase the risk of vision loss and blindness. Smoking when pregnant increases the risk of premature delivery, chances of birth defects

Smoking and tobacco use leads to disease and disability. It harms almost every organ in the body.

like cleft lip, cleft palate, or both in the newborn, breathing disorders in the newborn, slow development, and increases the chances of sudden infant death syndrome (SIDS).

Indirect consequences: Alcohol and drug misuse are linked to risky behaviors, as they can impair judgment. DUI is a major cause of accidents and accident-related deaths. Driving under the influence of alcohol or drugs contributes to thousands of deaths annually, and 10.6 percent of drivers report engaging in this hazardous behavior each year. Alcohol and drug misuse also increases the chances of HIV transmission caused by unprotected sex and sharing of needles/syringes.

Long-term consequences: Heavy drinking can lead to hypertension, liver disease, and cancer. Smoking and marijuana use is associated with chronic bronchitis, and the use of stimulants, such as cocaine, can lead to heart disease. Also, drug and alcohol use can lead to reduced productivity, higher healthcare costs, unintended pregnancies, the spread of infectious disease, drug-related crime, interpersonal violence, stress within families, and many other direct and indirect effects on communities, the economy, and society.

As per studies done in 2015, substance use disorders affected 20.8 million Americans, which is eight percent of the adolescent and adult population. This number is similar to the number of people who have diabetes and more than 1.5 times the annual prevalence of all cancers combined (14 million). Of the 20.8 million people with a substance use disorder in 2015, 15.7 million needed treatment for an alcohol problem and nearly 7.7 million needed treatments for an illicit drug problem.

I strongly recommend getting professional help if you have any addictions. Also, you may visit the reference links mentioned below to educate yourself and get some tips on how to quit smoking.

References:

- *U.S. Department of Health and Human Services. (n.d.). ALCOHOL AND TOBACCO. National Institute on Alcohol Abuse and Alcoholism. https://pubs.niaaa.nih.gov/publications/aa71/aa71.htm.*
- *Myers, M. G., & Kelly, J. F. (1970, January 1). Cigarette Smoking Among Adolescents With Alcohol and Other Drug Use Problems. Alcohol Research & Health. https://www.ncbi.nlm.nih.gov/pmc/articles/PMC1931414/.*
- *Sidebar: The Many Consequences of Alcohol and Drug Misuse. Sidebar: The Many Consequences of Alcohol and Drug Misuse | Surgeon General's Report on Alcohol, Drugs, and Health. (n.d.). https://addiction.surgeongeneral.gov/sidebar-many-consequences-alcohol-and-drug-misuse.*
- *Tips. Smokefree. (n.d.). https://smokefree.gov/tips.*
- *Centers for Disease Control and Prevention. (2020, November 16). Office on Smoking and Health (OSH). Centers for Disease Control and Prevention. https://www.cdc.gov/tobacco/about/osh/index.htm.*

CHAPTER 16

The Harmful Effects of Sugar and Artificial Sweeteners

KKK

S ugar and artificial sweeteners can cause serious havoc on our health. Hence, this chapter is very important so that we can understand the harmful effects of sugar and artificial sweeteners and discover better alternatives.

Let's review 10 main reasons to avoid sugar and a few tips on how to reduce sugar intake:

- Sugar can cause weight gain. Obesity is on the rise, and it has been found that the increase in sugar consumption is directly proportional to obesity. Sugary drinks, like juices and sodas, are responsible for this. These drinks do not provide any nutritional value and contain lots of empty calories. Also, they are full of fructose, and excessive consumption of fructose, which is a type of monosaccharide, may cause leptin resistance. Leptin is a hormone that signals your brain to stop eating. Leptin resistance disrupts this function, causing us to overeat. Eating fruits high in fructose is completely fine, as, in fruits, fructose occurs in its natural form, while in sodas, it is processed and has no nutritional value. Also, fruits have fiber and other nutrients, along with fructose, but drinking juices or sodas, which have nothing but fructose, is not recommended.

- Overconsumption of sugar can lead to an increased risk of heart disease. High-sugar diets can increase inflammation and blood sugar levels. This, in turn, increases the risk of heart disease.

- High-sugar diets, and foods with a high glycemic index, are the major cause of type 2 diabetes. These kinds of diets can cause obesity and insulin resistance in our bodies.

Overconsumption of sugar can lead to an increased risk of heart disease. High-sugar diets can increase inflammation and blood sugar levels.

- Too much sugar can cause acne and other skin-related problems. Too much consumption of sugar causes inflammation and spikes in blood sugar levels. These increase the secretion of the hormone androgen in the body. This results in the overproduction of sebum (oil) in the body. Sebum is responsible for clogged pores, resulting in acne.

- Diets high in sugar may increase wrinkles and speed up the aging of your skin. When we consume a diet high in sugar and/or foods with a high glycemic index, the production of compounds called advanced glycation end products (AGEs) increases in our bodies. AGEs are harmful free radicals that are responsible for damaging collagen and other proteins that help our skin maintain a youthful appearance.

- Excess sugar speeds up the aging process of our bodies. We must understand how the aging process works. At the end of our chromosomes, there are structures called telomeres, which act as a protective cap. As a natural process, telomeres become shorter and shorter, which causes our cells to age. Unhealthy food choices and lifestyle choices will speed up the shortening of telomeres, which, in turn, speeds up the aging process.

- Drains your energy. Diet high in sugar, or with a high glycemic index, will give sugar spikes, followed by a crash, which, in turn, will impact our energy levels.

- Sugar causes fatty liver and liver damage. Especially fructose from high-fructose corn syrup, which increases the risk of liver damage. Fructose is digested in our liver. Fructose from any fruit reaches our liver slowly, as our digestive system slowly processes it due to its fiber content. But, when we consume large amounts of processed fructose in the form of chemicals (synthetic sweeteners), or as high-fructose corn syrup, particularly in liquid form, it is processed by our digestive system vary rapidly due to the lack of fiber. This causes overload on our liver. This is the major cause of liver damage and fatty liver.

- Increase in the risk of gout and other inflammatory diseases.

- Harmful to your teeth and gums. Bacteria in our mouth thrive on sugar and releases acid byproducts, which will cause cavities.

In short, consuming a natural source of sugar is better for health than consuming added sugars or processed sugar.

Here are a few tips on reducing sugar intake:

- Swap sugary drinks and sodas for water or unsweetened seltzer.

- Swap store-bought yogurts with plain yogurt topped with fruits and honey or organic maple syrup.
- Be a vigilant shopper and read labels carefully. Watch out for added sugar. Here are some of the different names of sugar for your knowledge: anhydrous dextrose, brown sugar, confectioner's powdered sugar, corn syrup, corn syrup solids, dextrose, fructose, high-fructose corn syrup (HFCS), invert sugar, malt syrup, maltose, maple syrup, molasses, nectars (e.g., peach nectar, pear nectar), raw sugar, sucrose, white granulated sugar, cane juice, evaporated corn sweetener, crystal dextrose, glucose, liquid fructose, sugar cane juice, fruit nectar.
- Make your granola at home with honey or maple syrup and dates instead of buying store-bought ones.
- Top your bread with nut butter and fresh banana or strawberries instead of jams and jellies.
- Eat one to two dates or other fresh fruits instead of sugary desserts or candies.
- Use nut butter instead of Nutella on your bread.
- Do not buy packaged food if it contains more than four grams of sugar per serving.
- Consume fresh fruits instead of fruit juice or smoothies, which have added sugar.
- Do not consume alcoholic beverages that have sugar in them.

Now that we have reviewed the harmful effects of sugar and know that sugar is not good for us, what is the solution? Humans have been trying to satisfy our sweet tooth for centuries now, so, with the rise of diabetes and obesity, we have tried to come up with a solution, thinking that if a sweetener has zero calories, it is better than sugar. Guess what? We were absolutely wrong.

Artificial sweeteners are more harmful than sugar. The first

Artificial sweeteners are more harmful than sugar.

artificial sweetener invented was saccharin. I remember that many people with diabetes were thrilled with this invention. If only they knew the story behind this product, they would not have agreed to use it. Saccharin's commercial name is Sweet'N Low. It is a petroleum derivative called toluene. It has harmful side effects and increases sugar cravings and cravings for food, thus increasing obesity and the risk of type 2 diabetes. Research shows saccharin is also a carcinogen in animal studies. Over and above saccharin, several other artificial sweeteners were introduced in the last 50–60 years or so.

- A sweetener known as sodium cyclamate gained popularity and was used in diet sodas and other products, but it was banned in 1970 due to its carcinogenic properties. It is still banned in the U.S., as well as other countries.
- Then came aspartame, sold as Equal and NutraSweet. The ingredients are aspartic acid and PKU (phenylalanine). People thought this was much healthier than sugar and saccharin, but studies showed that it increased the risk of obesity and diabetes. Several European countries have banned it. It is still sold in the U.S., but studies have proven that this product increases the risk of obesity and diabetes, so I would not recommend this to anyone.
- Then came acesulfame K, sold as Sunett. The possible long-term side effects of this sweetener are appetite loss, headache, mental confusion, serious impact on kidneys and liver, bronchitis, cancer, and visual disturbances.
- In the meantime, another sweetener called neotame was introduced. This product was almost the same chemical

composition as aspartame. The chemical composition of this one is aspartame 3,3-dimethylbutyl, a very harmful chemical. I would not recommend using this one either.

- Then Splenda and sucralose came onto the market. The story behind the invention of Splenda is quite interesting. Sucralose is an artificial sweetener and the commercial name of Sucralose is Splenda. It is derived from sugar by chemically modifying it so that it is 600 times sweeter than sugar and has no calories. Studies show it can lead to obesity, possible fluctuations of insulin and blood glucose levels, and can alter your gut microbiome. Splenda and sucralose, when heated, release chloropropanols, which are very harmful to us.

Before we go gaga over the reduced calories in artificial sweeteners, I want to clarify two points. The first point is that no matter how many calories these sweeteners help us cut from our food, the harmful effects are so much that these sweeteners are not worth giving a shot. The second point is that these sweeteners are not zero calories. FDA labeling laws are a bit tricky. If a product has fewer than 20 calories per serving or less than five grams of carbs, it is considered zero calories. Now, while these products have fewer than 20 calories per serving, so are allowed to be labeled as zero calories. When you make a dessert using these products, you are not going to add just one packet. You will probably add a cup or so. Hence, they are not zero-calorie sweeteners.

So, I would highly recommend reconsidering your choice before you add that packet of artificial sweetener into your body. Reconsider before you pour that diet soda, or regular soda, into your cup. Don't be disheartened. There are some better alternatives to sugar and these harmful artificial sweeteners that will satisfy your sweet tooth.

We already know that excessive added sugar is harmful to our health. As we have seen, a high intake of sugar can increase the risks of obesity, diabetes, cancer, and other health problems. Also, sugar is addictive, as it causes our brain to release dopamine, which leads to cravings and overeating. Now we know how sugar sneaks into our food, so we need to be extra vigilant while we shop, reading labels, as well as nutrition facts, before we purchase any packaged food.

Reconsider before you pour that diet soda, or regular soda, into your cup.

At the same time, artificial sweeteners are not healthy either. We humans have been very innovative when it comes to satisfying our sweet tooth. Some ideas are not healthy at all, but, at the same time, we do have a few better alternatives.

As we know that there are lots of harmful side effects from excessive added sugar and artificial sweeteners, we have always tried to find better alternatives.

Let's discuss better alternatives to processed sugar and harmful artificial sweeteners.

1. **Stevia:** Stevia is a natural sweetener extracted from a plant called *Stevia rebaudiana*. It has no side effects and is a zero-calorie sweetener. Studies have shown that it also has some health benefits, like lowering blood pressure, blood sugar levels, and insulin levels. Stevia also has antioxidant compounds like glycosides and stevioside. When purchasing Stevia, choose organic raw Stevia instead of a processed variety. Even though it is a zero-calorie sweetener, I recommend using it in moderation because, when we add it to a dessert, there are added calories that come from other macronutrients.

2. **Xylitol:** Xylitol is a sugar alcohol with a glycemic index that

is 10 times lower than sugar. It is not a zero-calorie sweetener, however. It has 2.4 calories per gm, which is 40 percent less than sugar, but it does not have any valuable nutrients, so these are considered empty calories. It does have a few health benefits, as it helps in the prevention of tooth decay. It does not increase blood sugar levels or insulin levels. Also, it acts like soluble fiber and thus supports gut bacteria. Studies have shown that it may help improve calcium absorption in our body, which can help in the prevention of osteoporosis.

3. **Erythritol:** Erythritol is another sugar alcohol and contains just five percent of the calories of sugar, along with 70 percent of the sweetness of sugar. Studies show that it may have minimal effect on blood sugar levels, as most of it is excreted via urine and is not absorbed in the small intestine. Use this in moderation because overconsumption might cause minor digestive issues, like flatulence, bloating, and diarrhea, mostly in children.

4. **Monk Fruit Extract:** Pure monk fruit extract is also a great natural alternative to sugar, as it has zero calories and zero carbs. I have used it in my coffee, and it does not have an aftertaste. It helps in controlling blood sugar levels and contains natural antioxidants (mogrosides).

5. **Yacon Syrup:** Pure Yacon syrup is extracted from the yacon plant. Organic, pure, unprocessed Yacon syrup is thick in consistency, sweet, and dark in color. It contains 40 percent to 50 percent fructooligosaccharides. Our body cannot digest these fructooligosaccharides, and, hence, yacon syrup contains one-third of the calories of regular sugar. Studies have shown this can help in weight loss, too, as it may decrease levels of the hunger hormone ghrelin. Hence, this can help in suppressing the appetite. Fructooligosaccharides support healthy gut bacteria and, therefore, improve overall gut health

and decrease the risk of diabetes. However, overconsumption can lead to minor digestive issues. One more thing to remember is that yacon syrup cannot be heated, as heat breaks down fructooligosaccharides, but you can add it to smoothies, overnight oats, or your coffee.

There are other natural sugars, which are not as good as the above-mentioned natural alternatives, but which are still better than sugar or artificial sweeteners.
Here is a brief introduction to those:

1. **Coconut Sugar:** Extracted from the sap of the coconut palm. Coconut sugar has nutrients like iron, zinc, calcium, potassium, and antioxidants. It is also high in inulin, which is a natural fiber. Due to this, it has a lower glycemic index than sugar but the same number of calories, and is very high in fructose, so it should be used only rarely.
2. **Honey:** This thick golden liquid, produced by honeybees, is rich in antioxidants and micronutrients. It helps lower LDL and triglycerides. It also helps increase HDL. Honey is also an anti-inflammatory and offers other health benefits, so it is a better alternative than sugar. However, it is high in fructose, so it should be used sparingly.
3. **Maple Syrup:** This thick liquid is produced from maple sap. It has a good amount of minerals, is rich in antioxidants, and has some anti-cancer benefits. Maple syrup has a lower glycemic index than sugar, so it is a better alternative than sugar, but it is still high in fructose.
4. **Blackstrap Molasses and Jaggery:** Both are produced by boiling down sugar cane juice. Molasses can also be made by boiling down sugar beet juice. Both natural alternatives contain

nutrients that can support bone health and heart health. They may also help regulate blood sugar levels, but they are still high in sugar, so they should be consumed sparingly. I prefer raw, unprocessed, organic jaggery over molasses.

5. **Dates:** Dates are nutrient-dense fruit with several health benefits. They are high in several nutrients, fiber, and antioxidants, which may provide health benefits ranging from improved digestion to a reduced risk of diseases. You can eat them as a snack or add them to desserts. They are still high in calories (100 grams of dates equals 277 calories), so you might want to limit yourself to a few.

In summary, eating too much sugar is linked to several diseases, so I recommend substituting the above-mentioned natural sweeteners in your dishes instead of sugar, but at the same time, you should use them in moderation. Also, if you are watching calories for any reason, you must consider the total calories of that dish before you indulge too much in the desert.

Be very mindful about what you eat and plan your meals properly. If you plan to eat dessert, avoid carbs in the main course. Also, pair up the dessert with a big bowl of green salad and add some protein to the meal. This will add fiber and protein to your meal and reduce the glycemic index of the meal. Proper planning prevents poor performance. Also, eat desserts in moderation, keeping them for special occasions. As my dad used to say, anything in excess is poison.

References:

- *Dietary Guidelines for Americans. (2016, March). Cut Down On Added Sugars. Available from:* <u>https://www.nhlbi.nih.gov/news/2016/new-dietary-guidelines-urge-americans-eat-less-added-sugars-saturated-fat-and-sodium</u>
- *Trasande L, Shaffer RM, Sathyanarayana S; COUNCIL ON ENVIRONMENTAL HEALTH. Food Additives and Child Health. Pediatrics. 2018 Aug;142(2):e20181410. doi: 10.1542/peds.2018-1410. PMID: 30037972; PMCID: PMC6298598. Available from:* <u>https://www.ncbi.nlm.nih.gov/pmc/articles/PMC6298598/</u>
- *DiNicolantonio, J. J., Lucan, S. C., & O'Keefe, J. H. (2016). The Evidence for Saturated Fat and for Sugar Related to Coronary Heart Disease. Progress in cardiovascular diseases, 58(5), 464–472. Available from:* <u>https://pubmed.ncbi.nlm.nih.gov/26586275/</u>
- *Wang, M., Yu, M., Fang, L., & Hu, R. Y. (2015). Association between sugar-sweetened beverages and type 2 diabetes: A meta-analysis. Journal of diabetes investigation, 6(3), 360–366. Available from:* <u>https://www.ncbi.nlm.nih.gov/pmc/articles/PMC4420570/</u>
- *Schiffman, S. S., & Rother, K. I. (2013). Sucralose, a synthetic organochlorine sweetener: an overview of biological issues. Journal of toxicology and environmental health. Part B, Critical reviews, 16(7), 399–451. Available from:* <u>https://www.ncbi.nlm.nih.gov/pmc/articles/PMC3856475/</u>
- *Pepino MY, Tiemann CD, Patterson BW, Wice BM, Klein S. Sucralose affects glycemic and hormonal responses to an oral glucose load. Diabetes Care. 2013 Sep;36(9):2530-5. doi: 10.2337/dc12-2221. Epub 2013 Apr 30. PMID: 23633524; PMCID: PMC3747933. Available from:* <u>https://pubmed.ncbi.nlm.nih.gov/23633524/</u>

- *Ma J, Bellon M, Wishart JM, Young R, Blackshaw LA, Jones KL, Horowitz M, Rayner CK. Effect of the artificial sweetener, sucralose, on gastric emptying and incretin hormone release in healthy subjects. Am J Physiol Gastrointest Liver Physiol. 2009 Apr;296(4):G735-9. doi: 10.1152/ajpgi.90708.2008. Epub 2009 Feb 12. PMID: 19221011; PMCID: PMC2670679. Available from: https://pubmed.ncbi.nlm.nih.gov/19221011/*

- *Ma J, Chang J, Checklin HL, Young RL, Jones KL, Horowitz M, Rayner CK. Effect of the artificial sweetener, sucralose, on small intestinal glucose absorption in healthy human subjects. Br J Nutr. 2010 Sep;104(6):803-6. doi: 10.1017/S0007114510001327. Epub 2010 Apr 27. PMID: 20420761. Available from: https://pubmed.ncbi.nlm.nih.gov/20420761/*

- *Vazquez-Prieto, M. A., Rodriguez Lanzi, C., Lembo, C., Galmarini, C. R., & Miatello, R. M. (2011). Garlic and onion attenuates vascular inflammation and oxidative stress in fructose-fed rats. Journal of nutrition and metabolism, 2011, 475216. https://pubmed.ncbi.nlm.nih.gov/21876795/.*

CHAPTER 17

Harmful Effects of Preservatives, Artificial Colors, Artificial Flavors, Chemical Fertilizers, Pesticides, and GMOs

T his is a vast topic, and a whole book could be written about these harmful substances, but I will try my best to educate you on the adverse effect of chemicals on your health.

Preservatives are the chemical substances added to foods to increase their shelf life, while food colors and artificial flavors are added chemicals that enhance the appearance and taste of foods. The problem with all these substances is that they are chemicals made in factories. Our bodies are not well-equipped to absorb, digest, and process the chemicals, but the modern food industry is trying to turn our bodies into chemical factories so that they can sell more products, get us addicted to their junk food, and make more profits. Keep one thing in mind: "The greater the shelf life, the less your life."

Let's check out the history of artificial food colors. Food manufacturers have been using artificial food colors for ages. Years ago, they were created from coal tar, and, in modern days, they are made from petroleum. Now, before you reach for that bag of chips and before you give your kids those colorful candies, close your eyes and visualize serving yourself or your children petroleum on a platter to eat. If you wouldn't do that, stop eating it in junk food simply because it tastes good. Most artificial food colorings are highly toxic, and they are the primary cause of chronic inflammation in our bodies. Some food manufacturers use natural colors, like beet extract or beta carotene, but most of them use artificial colors because they are cheaper than natural alternatives, and they give a more vibrant color.

Even though the U.S. Food and Drug Administration (FDA) and European Food Safety Authority (EFSA) have concluded that these dyes do not pose significant health risks, the research and studies have been done on animals and not on humans. Also, some food dyes are considered safe in one country while banned in another.

Here is a list of a few commonly used artificial colors:

- **Red No. 3 (erythrosine):** A cherry red dye. Used in candy, popsicles, and cake-decorating gels.
- **Red No. 40 (Allura Red):** A dark red dye. Used in sports drinks, candy, condiments, and cereals.
- **Yellow No. 5 (tartrazine):** A lemon yellow dye. Used in candy, soft drinks, chips, popcorn, and cereals.
- **Yellow No. 6 (Sunset Yellow):** An orange-yellow dye. Used in candy, sauces, baked goods, and preserved fruits.

- **Blue No. 1 (Brilliant Blue):** A greenish-blue dye. Used in ice cream, canned peas, packaged soups, popsicles, and icings.
- **Blue No. 2 (indigo carmine):** A royal blue dye. Used in candy, ice cream, cereal, and snacks.

Artificial food colors are highly toxic and can cause chronic inflammation, allergies, ADHD, and cancer. Preservatives and other chemicals found in food and other consumer goods that we use in our day-to-day lives also harm our health. Synthetic chemicals are used as food preservatives to increase the shelf life of food, enhance the flavor, and, to a certain extent, can make you addicted to that food. Most of these chemicals mess up your hormones. The most-used preservatives and flavor enhancers in foods are sodium benzoate, benzoic acid, sodium sorbate, potassium sorbate, sodium nitrite, and monosodium glutamate (MSG). As with artificial colors, these preservatives can cause chronic inflammation, hormonal imbalance, allergies, ADHD, cancer, heart disease, headaches, obesity, thyroid issues, skin rashes, asthma, nausea, etc.

Artificial food colors are highly toxic and can cause chronic inflammation, allergies, ADHD, and cancer.

There are natural ways to preserve food, including the use of sugar, oil, and salt, and through methods like fermentation, curing, jellying, dehydrating, and freezing. In Indian cooking, pickles have been made at home using oil, salt, and sugar, and these can last almost a year. I am not saying that these are super healthy because Indian pickles contain high amounts of oil, sugar, and salt, but they are better than food that has been preserved using chemicals.

In addition to these preservatives, we come across other chemicals in our day-to-day lives, which are found in consumer goods, like food cans, plastic bottles, skincare and body care products, nail polish, makeup, etc.

Here are a few of those chemicals and the harmful effects they cause:

- **Bisphenols, such as BPA:** Found in the lining of food and soda cans, plastics, and plastic bottles. These can act like the hormone estrogen and interfere with puberty and fertility. Bisphenols can also increase body fat and cause problems with the immune system and nervous system.
- **Phthalates:** These are found in personal-use products, like nail polish, hair sprays, body lotions, perfumes, etc. They are also found in plastic packaging, garden hoses, and some toys. These can also act like hormones, interfering with male genital development, and can increase the risk of obesity and cardiovascular disease.
- **Perfluoroalkyl chemicals (PFCs):** Commonly found in grease-proof paper, cardboard packaging, and commercial household products, such as water-repellent fabrics and nonstick pans. These can lead to low-birthweight babies, as well as problems with the immune system, thyroid, and fertility.
- **Perchlorate:** Found in dry-food packaging and sometimes in drinking water. This interferes with thyroid function and can disrupt early brain development.
- **Nitrates and nitrites:** Commonly found in processed foods and processed meats. These can interfere with the thyroid, as well as with the blood's ability to deliver oxygen to the body. They can also increase the risk of certain cancers.

Pesticides and fertilizers are the chemicals used in farming practices to protect crops and increase the quantity of crops. Excessive use of chemical fertilizers and pesticides is detrimental to human health, as well as the environment. These chemicals damage lungs and the nervous system. Some of them are carcinogens. Additionally, they increase water, air, and soil pollution. The "Dirty Dozen" is a trademarked term used to define the 12 crops that farmers typically use the most pesticides on, versus the "Clean 15," which is also a trademarked term to describe the 15 fruits and vegetables that have the lowest amount of pesticide residue. The Dirty Dozen vegetables and fruits, which absorb these chemicals easily, are recommended to be avoided in their non-organic versions at all costs. You can find a list of the Dirty Dozen here: https://www.ewg.org/foodnews/dirty-dozen.php

The "Dirty Dozen" is a trademarked term used to define the 12 crops that farmers typically use the most pesticides on, versus the "Clean 15," which is also a trademarked term to describe the 15 fruits and vegetables that have the lowest amount of pesticide residue.

One more thing you should consider is that if you consume meat, then you also consume whatever that animal was fed. If that animal was fed growth hormones, fattening foods, and antibiotics, all those harmful substances would end up in your body, causing havoc in your gut, which can lead to obesity, hormonal imbalance, and antibiotic resistance. In short, for a non-vegetarian person, your health not only depends on what you eat but also on what the animals you consume ate.

GMOs

GMO stands for a genetically modified organism, an organism whose gene pattern is altered in a way that does not occur naturally. Scientists alter the gene patterns of organisms, crops, or plants for several reasons, such as to increase the production of the crop or to make that crop disease resistant. This technology is often called "modern biotechnology," "gene technology," "recombinant DNA technology," or "genetic engineering."

While there is research going on about the impact of GMOs on human health, there are several controversies around GMOs. The major concern is the possibility that GMOs negatively affect human health in the form of an allergic response or with undesired side effects, such as toxicity, organ damage, or gene transfer.

We will discuss more about how you can avoid these chemicals in your food in Part II when we talk about nutrition and mindful eating. But, in short, consume foods that grow on plants, are all-natural, and free of any chemical additives. Stick to organic food, as some of the harmful chemicals (pesticides and fertilizers) used in farming practices are detrimental to our health.

You must read the nutrition labels of the foods you buy at the grocery store to ensure that they are free of artificial colors, preservatives, and artificial flavors. Read the ingredient lists on the labels of your skincare, makeup, and personal care products, to ensure they do not contain harmful chemicals.

Also, instead of plastic water bottles or store-bought water in plastic bottles, invest in a good-quality, at-home water filtration system, as these chemicals do sneak into your drinking water. Store food in glass containers instead of plastic ones. Take cloth or paper shopping bags with you so that you do not have to use the plastic bags provided by the store. You will help the environment by reducing plastic waste and improving the quality of your life, as well as your health.

References:

- Aktar, M. W., Sengupta, D., & Chowdhury, A. (2009). *Impact of pesticides use in agriculture: their benefits and hazards. Interdisciplinary toxicology, 2(1), 1–12. Available from:* https://www.ncbi.nlm.nih.gov/pmc/articles/PMC2984095/
- Bawa, A. S., & Anilakumar, K. R. (2013). *Genetically modified foods: safety, risks, and public concerns-a review. Journal of food science and technology, 50(6), 1035–1046. Available from:* https://www.ncbi.nlm.nih.gov/pmc/articles/PMC3791249/

PART II

"The doctor of the future will give no medicine, but will instruct his patients in the care of the human frame, in diet, and in the cause and prevention of disease." – Thomas Edison

CHAPTER 18

12 Steps to Optimal Well-Being

⫷⫷⫷

I n the previous section, we reviewed the meaning of optimal well-being and why we should strive for it, as well as several factors, like evidence-based functional and lifestyle medicine and hormones, in addition to lifestyle changes, which play an important role in achieving optimal well-being. We also understood circadian rhythms, unique mind-body constitution, and the importance of developing a daily routine.

In our next section, we will review the 12 steps to optimal well-being and their role in all aspects of well-being. In short, in Part I, we examined the "what" and "why" of optimal well-being, while in Part II, we shall review how a simple, 12-step program can help someone achieve optimal well-being in all the dimensions of life, such as physical, spiritual, social, intellectual, environmental, financial, mental, and emotional well-being. As we go to part II of this book, where you will learn the 12 steps to optimal well-being, visualize an orchestra in your mind. As several musicians come together and play all the instruments in harmony to create a beautiful symphony, in the same manner, all these 12 steps can create an amazing life for you.

The purpose of this book, as I mentioned earlier, is to help you in your quest for optimal well-being, as it is your birthright. Optimal well-being is our innate nature, and when we live in harmony with the universe, we achieve it effortlessly. Ayurveda recommends to be mindful about aahar(food), vihar (movement) and vichar (thoughts) to maintain your aarogya (well-being). We must always remember that whatever we focus on grows, so it is essential to think right. A healthy mind will mirror the thoughts of wellness, while illness will manifest in the body if we are afraid of getting sick. Optimal well-being is a vast subject, so I understand that it might become overwhelming to comprehend, but I assure you that, by the time you are done with this book, you will be able to understand the subject, as well as define your path toward optimal well-being.

I strongly encourage you to

As we go to part II of this book, where you will learn the 12 steps to optimal well-being, visualize an orchestra in your mind. As several musicians come together and play all the instruments in harmony to create a beautiful symphony, in the same manner, all these 12 steps can create an amazing life for you.

Ayurveda recommends to be mindful about aahar (food), vihar (movement) and vichar (thoughts) to maintain your aarogya (well-being).

take note of your thoughts and feelings and to journal them as you read. Also, remember that sometimes it is overwhelming if we try to make drastic changes in our lifestyle, but change becomes easy when we take small steps. Hence, it is important to set *SMART* goals (to be discussed in detail in a later chapter) when working on making lifestyle changes. Throughout Part II, we shall talk more about taking baby steps toward improvement and being mindful, as mindfulness is the key. It is important to listen to your body while you are making changes, incorporating what works for you, and leaving the rest.

Throughout the book, I have been emphasizing mindfulness, so you might be wondering, What does being mindful mean? Mindfulness means living in the present and being aware of what is happening in the current moment. Learning to be mindful is highly beneficial for our overall well-being, and this skill can be easily acquired with practice.

Most of the time in our lives, we are on autopilot. Multitasking is considered highly efficient in the modern world, but it is not a fact. Many people eat while reading, watching TV, attending meetings, or thinking and worrying about the future, so they end up not enjoying the taste of their meals, nor do they enjoy the company of friends and family members who may be with them at the dining table. This also leads to overeating. I have also noticed people exercising while watching TV or a movie instead of being in tune with their bodies. This can lead to overexerting a certain muscle group resulting in injury.

Mindfulness is a way to break free from this robotic lifestyle. It teaches us to pay attention to our thoughts, feelings, behaviors, and habits without being judgmental. It allows us to pause, enjoy the moment, and reflect on the choices we can make that will assist us toward improving our future. Mindfulness teaches us to notice our emotions when we are in an unpleasant situation and helps us reflect on our thoughts and respond to the situation in a stable state of mind, instead of just reacting to it. Hence, mindfulness is an important skill, and everyone should acquire it.

As Thich Nhat Hanh says, "Mindfulness shows us what is happening in our bodies, our emotions, our minds, and in the world. Through mindfulness, we avoid harming ourselves and others."

"Breathing in, I am aware that I am breathing in.
Breathing out, I am aware that I am breathing out.
Breathing in, I am grateful for this moment.
Breathing out, I smile.
Breathing in, I am aware of the preciousness of this day.
Breathing out, I vow to live deeply in this day."

- Thich Nhat Hanh

CHAPTER 19

Step 1: Deep Restful Sleep

"A good laugh and a long sleep are the best cures in the doctor's book." — *Irish Proverb.*

निद्रायत्तं सुखं दुःखं पुष्टिः कार्श्यं बलाबलम् वृषता क्लीबता
ज्ञानमज्ञानं जीवितं न च३६
अकालेऽतिप्रसङ्गाच्च न च निद्रा निषेविता सुखायुषी पराकुर्यात्
कालरात्रिरिवापरा३७
सैव युक्ता पुनर्युङ्क्ते निद्रा देहं सुखायुषा पुरुषं योगिनं सिद्ध्या
सत्या बुद्धिरिवागता३८

In human beings, happiness and misery, nourishment and emaciation, strength and weakness, fertility and infertility, knowledge and ignorance, and longevity and death depend upon proper (and improper sleep). Untimely, excessive sleep and sleep deprivation take away both happiness and longevity from a person. Similarly, proper sleep brings about happiness and longevity in human beings just as real knowledge brings about spiritual power in yogis. - Charak Samhita

I believe that deep, restful sleep is the first step to attaining optimal well-being. In India, sleep is also referred to as "Nidrā Devī" where "Devi" means "Goddess" and "Nidrā" means "Sleep." Research says that adults need between seven and nine hours of sleep at night, and sleep is a highly essential part of our daily routine. But the quality of sleep is equally important. Getting the right amount of sleep at the right time is as essential as food and water. Your productivity during the day and the quality of your day will depend on how well you slept the previous night.

Maintaining proper sleep hygiene is important for optimal brain functions, as it improves our brain's ability to learn new things, concentrate, and respond. Over and above that, sleep supports communication between our nerve cells and between the cells of different parts of our bodies. Even when we are sleeping, our brain and body stay active to remove toxins, restore, repair, and rejuvenate.

Hence, we all need adequate sleep, as it impacts the health of every tissue and cell in our bodies, from the brain, heart, immune function, and lungs. It also impacts our metabolism, and several studies have shown that lack of sleep, or poor-quality sleep, is a major cause of obesity, hypertension, cardiovascular diseases, depression, increased stress, inflammation, and diabetes. During deep sleep, your body releases accumulated stress and physical toxins, balances hormones, strengthens the immune system, and repairs and regenerates cells and tissues.

We will not go into detail about the anatomy of sleep in this chapter, but we shall review the stages of sleep and how you can develop a healthy sleep routine in harmony with circadian rhythms to gain optimal benefit.

The two types of sleep are REM and non-REM sleep. Each of these is connected to specific brain activity. When we sleep at night, we all go through the stages of REM and non-REM sleep several times during the night. Each cycle lasts for about ninety minutes and continues throughout the night. The first ninety minutes after falling asleep is non-REM sleep, which is divided into three stages, as explained below.

Stage 1 is non-REM sleep, which moves from wakefulness to sleep. This is a short period, which consists of relatively light sleep, where your heartbeat, breathing, and eye moments are slowing down. Your muscles have started to relax, and brain waves begin to slow down as well.

Stage 2 is also a non-REM sleep, which is the light sleep right before you enter deep sleep. Your heartbeat and breathing slow down further, and your muscles completely relax. Body temperature drops, and eye movement stops. Brain activity is very slow.

Stage 3, another non-REM sleep, is deep sleep. You need deep sleep to feel refreshed in the morning, and it is difficult to awaken you during deep sleep. If you wake up during this period, you will feel very groggy. This deep sleep occurs for a longer period during the first half of the night. Your heartbeat and breathing are at their lowest level.

Stage 4, or first REM sleep, occurs about ninety minutes after falling asleep. Most of our dreaming is during the REM sleep cycle. Our eyes move rapidly behind closed eyelids, breathing becomes faster, and heart rate and blood pressure increase. Your eyes move rapidly from side to side, behind closed eyelids. Mixed-frequency brain wave activity becomes similar to one when you are awake. Your breathing becomes faster and irregular, and your heart rate and blood pressure increase to near waking levels. Memory consolidation most likely requires both non-REM and REM sleep.

Thus, throughout the night, you alternate between ninety-minute cycles of non-REM and REM sleep, and the duration of REM sleep decreases near morning time.

In Chapter 12, we learned about circadian rhythms and the importance of maintaining a healthy routine in harmony with the rhythms of nature. We learned that it is important to go to bed by 10 p.m. so that our body clock is aligned with the circadian rhythm. We also learned that 10 p.m. to 2 a.m. is the "repair and restore" time. During this pitta time, our body is effectively metabolizing everything we ingest through our five senses, converting it into vital energy while discarding the waste and toxins. Our body's efficiency in repairing and restoring is at an optimal level when we are asleep by 10 p.m. This is the time when we get the best sleep quality.

For some people, if they wake up between 2 a.m. and 6 a.m., it becomes difficult for them to fall asleep again. That is because this is vata time, as per Ayurveda. During this time, vata dominates the environment, as well as our nervous system, due to which our mind becomes very active. People with a vata dosha predominance already have a busy or overactive mind, which can quickly become overactive or anxious, making falling asleep again very difficult.

In short, if you are feeling drowsy during the day, or if you are waking up feeling tired, your sleep pattern is probably to blame. If you have chronic inflammation, lifestyle-related illnesses, stress, anxiety, depression, slow metabolism, or difficulty losing weight even with eating the proper diet and exercising, you need to improve your sleep hygiene.

In short, if you are feeling drowsy during the day, or if you are waking up feeling tired, your sleep pattern is probably to blame.

Here are a few tips to improve the quality of sleep:

- Drink warm milk, soothing herbal tea, or a turmeric latte before bedtime.
- Try using natural, non-habit-forming sleep aids, like chamomile, lavender, etc.
- Take a warm bubble bath before bedtime.
- Say no to technology one to two hours before bed. If you are mentally stimulated, it will be difficult to fall asleep.
- Say no to caffeine after 6 p.m.
- Try self-massage with warm, soothing oils.
- Experiment with aromatherapy. Scents like lavender, chamomile, ylang-ylang oil, valerian oil, jasmine oil may improve the quality of your sleep.
- Relax with music or sounds of nature.
- Eat a light dinner at least two to three hours before bedtime because undigested food in the gut will prevent you from falling asleep or staying asleep.
- Go for a gentle walk for 15 to 20 minutes after meals to aid with digestion.
- Read a self-help book or personal development book before bedtime.
- Meditation helps to calm you down and enhances the quality of sleep.
- Remain physically active throughout the day so that your body is tired at night, but try to exercise before early evening because exercise will energize you. If you exercise right before bedtime, you will have difficulty falling asleep.
- Maintain a comfortable room temperature, around 67 degrees F. A room that is too cold or too hot will not facilitate optimal sleep.

- Try journaling, as it helps to process thoughts, emotions, and events of the day.
- Maintain a gratitude journal so that you can stay positive and calm.
- Once in bed, close your eyes, tune in to your body and breath, and quickly fall asleep.

I encourage you to come up with more ideas and journal them for future reference.

References:

- *Chopra, D. D., Kshirsagar, D. S., Simon, D. D., Patel, D. S., Porter, D. V., Saint, D. M., Gabriel, R., Stern, E., & Nadarajah, M. (2019, November). The perfect health ayurvedic lifestyle online enrichment program. Session 1 - 15.*
- *U.S. Department of Health and Human Services. (n.d.). Brain Basics: Understanding Sleep. National Institute of Neurological Disorders and Stroke. https://www.ninds.nih.gov/Disorders/Patient-Caregiver-Education/Understanding-Sleep.*

CHAPTER 20

Step 2: Detoxification

⋘⋘

"What's the most effective detox program?
Distancing yourself from self-destructive thoughts,
behaviors, and people." — *Charles F Glassman*

Detoxification is a treatment intended to remove poisonous or harmful substances, which can also be called ama or toxins, from our body. Our body is highly intelligent and has a natural ability to heal itself, but the problem is we get in its way. Due to our current fast and stressful lifestyle, our body and mind are in a constant state of stress. Hence, we experience chronic inflammation, which results in lifestyle-related illnesses and conditions.

Modern medicine doesn't have all the answers regarding diseases related to chronic inflammation or diseases that occur due to poor lifestyle choices. Whenever I see an advertisement for any prescription drug, it has more side effects than benefits. The height of insanity is that the side effects of antidepressant medication may increase suicidal thoughts. It is also greatly upsetting that modern medicine does not know the food industry, while the food industry does not care about our health. There is a huge disconnection between the two.

According to Ayurveda, most lifestyle-related illnesses and conditions are due to chronic inflammation and the accumulation of toxins in our body, produced by our poor lifestyle choices. As we saw in Chapter 10, if we have a healthy metabolism, our body will produce vital energy (ojas) from whatever we consume through our five senses. When our body is not able to properly metabolize the food we eat, the liquids we intake, and the experiences we encounter, it produces toxins (ama).

Toxins are created in our body due to several reasons: a poor diet; consumption of junk food full of artificial colors, preservatives, artificial flavors, and chemicals; consumption of sugar and unhealthy fats; overconsumption of salt; consumption of processed food; lack of sleep; use of synthetic chemicals in our diet; harsh chemicals in our home care products; chemicals in our skincare products, cosmetics, and environment; poorly digested food; environmental stress and fatigue; pollution; anxiety; anger; self-criticism; negativity; etc.

Fortunately, our body is highly capable of getting rid of accumulated toxins daily, but we can get in its way with our reckless lifestyle. No matter how careful we are, our body will produce some toxins daily, which we eliminate as waste through sweat, urine, and stool, but when these toxins are produced in excess, they start blocking the channels of elimination. When we don't change our habits, we produce toxins at a faster rate than our bodies can eliminate. These toxins enter our bloodstream and are transported to other organs of our body through the circulatory system. Slowly but surely, they find a weak spot in our body and start accumulating there, causing chronic inflammation.

Now, there is a difference between acute inflammation and chronic low-level inflammation. Acute inflammation is necessary for our body to heal. For example, if we have a cut on our finger, we experience acute, localized inflammation in that area. Blood rushes to the injured part, carrying platelets to form a clot so that excess bleeding will stop, and the cut can heal. As for chronic inflammation, it is the leading cause of lifestyle-related illnesses and conditions like diabetes, autoimmune diseases, cancer, arthritis, coronary artery disease, high blood pressure, digestive disorders, compromised immunity, and many more.

Chronic inflammation and the accumulation of toxins play a major role in autoimmune disorders. Our immune system views these toxins as a threat and becomes activated. These toxins also weaken our immune system and, as these toxins accumulate in our tissues and organs, our immune system attacks that part of our body.

Our immune system views these toxins as a threat and becomes activated. These toxins also weaken our immune system and, as these toxins accumulate in our tissues and organs, our immune system attacks that part of our body.

We must keep in mind the importance of reducing chronic inflammation by removing accumulated toxins, through detoxification, and adapting to a healthier lifestyle to reduce further production of toxins. Detoxification is an important step toward optimal well-being, as it improves physical and emotional well-being. A healthy body and healthy mind are vital for social well-being, as well as to improve productivity and performance at work.

Here are a few tips on how to facilitate daily detoxification:

- Early autumn and early spring are the perfect time to do a gentle detox so that you can reset your metabolism.
- Intermittent fasting is the best way to improve metabolism and remove toxins, but it does not work well for everyone. Hence, we must know more about Ayurvedic body types, like intermittent fasting (IF) works great for people who are kapha types, as they have a very slow and sluggish metabolism, and they respond very well to intermittent fasting. Normally, the 16:8 ratio (16 hours of fasting and eating during an 8-hour window) works best for them. Both pitta and vata types also should do fasting because no one should bombard their digestive organs with food all the time, but, in their case, a 12:12 ratio can work better.
- During detox, one should restrict themselves to 3 light easy to digest meals a day and sip warm liquids and warm caffeine-free herbal teas throughout the day to gently ignite their digestive fire.
- One more way to detox is by doing a juice detox or a liquid detox, where one consumes just clear liquids or juices from vegetables and fruits for a period of three to seven days to give rest to their digestive system and remove toxins. But a juice detox or IF is not for everyone. Hence, another way of doing a gentle detox is by incorporating certain Ayurvedic routines in our daily schedule, as mentioned in Chapter 13 and Chapter 14.
- Adding cleansing vegetables, like dandelion greens, kale, spinach, chard, collard greens, cucumbers, capsicum (peppers), bottle gourd, bitter gourd, green apples, red cabbage, celery, lemon, blueberries, cranberries, strawberries, kiwi, watercress, wheatgrass, ginger, celery, or turmeric root, to your juice or

smoothies during a juice detox or IF, or start your day with juice or smoothies that contain these vegetables and fruits as a great way to do a detox and also give your body a healthy dose of vitamins, minerals, phytonutrients, antioxidants, and fiber.

- Herbs like Triphala, milk thistle, fiber, and probiotics may help with a gentle detox.

- Starting your day with the juice of half a lemon and one tablespoon of honey in warm water helps to detox your system. If you have sluggish digestion, which is true for people with excess kapha dosha, you can add a tablespoon of fresh ginger juice, a pinch of salt, and a pinch of black pepper powder to this.

- Consuming light and easy-to-digest foods for a week, like clear soups made with cleansing vegetables like spinach, kale, chard, cauliflower, cabbage, broccoli, ginger, garlic, onions, red chilies or paprika, and turmeric, or consuming khichdi or moong bean soup, will give rest to your digestive system and help with a gentle detox. I prefer warm soups in the fall and winter and juices and smoothies in the summer.

- Use a tongue scraper and oil pulling first thing in the morning. This is the most effective way to get rid of toxins from your tongue and mouth. There are more than 10,000 taste buds on your tongue. By removing the toxins from the tongue and mouth, you will improve the capabilities of your taste buds. Food will taste better, and you will not need extra salt or sugar.

- Consume a lot of leafy greens, fibrous vegetables. Include greens like mustard greens, spinach, dandelion greens, arugula, lettuce, spinach, etc., in your diet, all of which have a mildly bitter flavor. The fiber, water, bitter taste, and nutrients in leafy green vegetables stimulate detoxification and digestion.

- Try dry skin brushing and oil massage. These techniques will help to increase the circulation of the lymphatic system.

Many toxins are in our lymphatic system and with the help of dry brushing and abhyanga (oil massage), we can get rid of these toxins.

- Increase water consumption and stay hydrated. Water will help your body get rid of toxins through urine.
- Exercise and use a steam sauna or dry sauna. In short, make sure that you sweat every day. Our skin is the largest organ in our body, and when we sweat, not only do we help our body to regulate its temperature, but we also help our body to eliminate toxins.
- Get a good night's sleep. When we rest, our bodies heal.
- Practice yoga and pranayama. Deep breathing techniques, called pranayama, is a gentle method to eliminate toxins from your airways and lungs.
- Limit the intake of toxins while trying to eliminate toxins from your body. To achieve this, eliminate processed food, excess salt, sugar, artificial sweeteners, food coloring and preservatives, flavor enhancers, alcohol, etc., from your diet.
- Switch to green products in your house as much as possible. Switch to more natural alternatives from your regular cleaning products, which are loaded with chemicals. This removes toxins from your environment and improves the quality of your surroundings.
- Say no to smoking, tobacco use, and substance abuse.
- Invest in a good-quality water purification system. Remember lead poisoning in the drinking water of Flint, Michigan, in 2014, which adversely impacted the health of thousands of people? Yes, be extra vigilant about your drinking water, as there are high chances that your drinking water may contain contaminants and chemical pollutants.
- While we are eliminating toxins from our bodies, it is also

important to eliminate toxins from our minds and environment to reduce environmental and mental stress. Hence, refrain from watching the news, television, or movies first thing in the morning or right before bedtime. Along with intermittent fasting, go for a technology fast. Say no to negativity, gossip, complaining and criticizing, anger, and jealousy for your emotional and mental well-being. Go on a gossip detox to improve your social well-being.

- Start your day right with a morning meditation.
- Find ways to express gratitude for the things you have, experiences in life, people around you, and your loved ones. A genuine feeling of gratitude leads to a happy and healthy heart.
- Develop a sleep routine to facilitate great sleep. A well-rested body and mind can function well and heal faster. Don't use technology before at least one hour before bedtime. Avoid eating at least three to four hours before bedtime. Avoid caffeine, or any mental stimulants, before bedtime. Wind down before sleep by turning off the lights. Listen to calming, relaxing music. Manage stress well.
- Ayurvedic panchakarma treatment mentioned in Part I of this book is also a great way to remove toxins from your body and heal it at a cellular level.
- Finally, laugh a lot. Laughter is the best medicine. Have fun, learn to live in the moment, and have a light heart.

I encourage you to write down in a journal some more detoxification ideas that would work for you.

References:

- *Chopra, D. D., Kshirsagar, D. S., Simon, D. D., Patel, D. S., Porter, D. V., Saint, D. M., Gabriel, R., Stern, E., & Nadarajah, M. (2019, November). The perfect health ayurvedic lifestyle online enrichment program. Session 1–15.*

- *Peterson CT, Denniston K, Chopra D. Therapeutic Uses of Triphala in Ayurvedic Medicine. J Altern Complement Med. 2017 Aug;23(8):607-614. doi: 10.1089/acm.2017.0083. Epub 2017 Jul 11. PMID: 28696777; PMCID: PMC5567597. Available from: https://pubmed.ncbi.nlm.nih.gov/28696777/*

- *Hodges, R. E., & Minich, D. M. (2015). Modulation of Metabolic Detoxification Pathways Using Foods and Food-Derived Components: A Scientific Review with Clinical Application. Journal of nutrition and metabolism, 2015, 760689. https://www.ncbi.nlm.nih.gov/pmc/articles/PMC4488002/*

CHAPTER 21

Step 3: Nutrition and Mindful Eating

"If the diet is wrong, medicine is of no use. If the diet is correct, medicine is of no need." – Ancient Ayurvedic proverb.

As you read earlier in the book, my journey in search of some answers related to my wellness started with the course in nutrition and healthy living. After some introspection and realization, I was led to Ayurveda. The more I learned, the more I was inspired to keep learning and growing, which led me to this point in my life where I have been able to summarize my knowledge about optimal well-being into 12 simple steps. Nutrition and mindful eating are some of the most important steps to attain physical as well as emotional well-being.

I am sure that now you know that well-being and weight loss

depend not only on the quantity of the calories but also on the quality of the calories. Calories from a good nutritious diet are not the same as calories from junk food. Even when two people living under one roof are consuming the same food, their wellness journey can be different because of several factors like hormones, individual mind-body constitution, stress levels, exercise habits, and sleep habits. My point is that the weight-loss or wellness journey of an individual is unique, and there is no cookie-cutter approach.

Also, several other factors, like hormones, metabolism, inflammation, digestion, basal metabolic rate, an individual's socio-economic environment, emotional wellness, sleep habits, stress level, etc., play an essential role. Hence, I started my journey to learn Ayurveda, hoping that my questions would be answered by this ancient wisdom.

The topic of mindful eating explains the significant difference between the science of conventional nutrition and ayurvedic nutrition in a very simple language. I hope this book will help readers make the right choices to support their optimal well-being. We all know that conventional nutrition focuses on counting calories and macronutrients. The importance is given to the caloric value, and the dietary advice focuses on food groups as it is believed that "you are what you eat." This is a great start for someone who has never focused on eating a healthy, nutrient-rich diet, but Ayurveda takes it a few steps further.

According to Ayurveda, you are what you digest. Ayurveda focuses on digestion, or digestive fire, also called digestive agni. Instead of caloric value, Ayurveda focuses on the individual constitution, and dietary advice depends on food quality and eating as per the individual constitution and taste. By understanding your unique mind-body constitution, you can choose foods that will nourish your body and help you reach a state of optimal well-being.

In Chapter 10, we understood the effects of a weak metabolism or weak digestive fire. If your digestive fire is balanced, your body will produce ojas (vitality) from whatever you consume through your five senses (food, liquids, air, touch, experiences, etc.), but if your digestive fire is weak or irregular, your body will produce ama (toxins) from whatever you consume.

By understanding your unique mind-body constitution, you can choose foods that will nourish your body and help you reach a state of optimal well-being.

As an illustration, imagine a wood-burning fireplace. If the fire is balanced, whatever you throw in will burn and get converted to heat and ashes. But, if the fire is weak or irregular, whatever you throw in will create lots of smoke and may extinguish the fire. And the same fire, when it is sharp, it gets out of control, can burn the whole house down. The same thing happens in your body.

A healthy balanced digestive fire will transform everything you consume into vitality and energy, while an unhealthy digestive fire will transform it into toxins.

The job of agni (digestive fire) in our body is to transform. A healthy balanced digestive fire will transform everything you consume into vitality and energy, while an unhealthy digestive fire will transform it into toxins.

Also, in Chapter 11, we learned about the unique mind-body constitution and different Ayurvedic body types. As a recap, vata type people have sensitive and irregular digestion. Pitta types have robust digestion and can digest anything easily, but, at the same time, if a pitta dosha becomes imbalanced, the same robust digestion can turn into very sharp agni similar to a wildfire and cause havoc in their system. Just like in a wood-burning fireplace, when the fire is burning at its peak, if you add too much oil or gasoline, it can cause too big of a fire. On the other hand, kapha types have very slow and sluggish digestion because they have weak agni. If they consume heavy meals, they are going to extinguish the agni. As an illustration, visualize that the wood in the fireplace is wet, and, hence, the fire is very weak and slow. If you add more heavy logs to this dim fire, it will extinguish.

Remember from Chapter 11 that the best way to maintain all the doshas in balance is to identify your unique mind-body constitution and then incorporate the principle of samanya (similarity) and vishesha (difference) in your diet. To recap, the similarity of all substances is always the cause of the increase, and the dissimilarity is the cause of the decrease.

As we learned in Part I, people with vata dosha predominance should minimize foods that are pungent, bitter, and astringent while incorporating foods that are sweet, salty, and sour. Also, to counterbalance the light, dry, cool properties of vata dosha, they should consume foods that are heavy, oily, and warm. People with pitta dosha predominance should consume foods that are sweet, bitter, and astringent in taste and minimize foods that are sour, salty, and pungent in taste. Also, to counterbalance the hot nature of the pitta dosha, ayurveda traditionally recommends foods that have a cooling effect. People with kapha dosha predominance should consume foods that are pungent, bitter, and astringent in taste and minimize foods that are sour, salty, and sweet. Also, to counterbalance the heavy and dull nature of the kapha dosha, Ayurveda traditionally recommends foods that are light, warm, and have a heating effect.

Instead of rushing through the meals or grabbing the bite on the go, learn to be a mindful eater. Focus on the taste and texture of the food. Ask yourself questions like, what do you like about that particular dish, how do you feel about the food choices you have made, how will it impact your health, are you really hungry, or are you bored? Mindful eating addresses three factors. What to eat, how to eat, and when to eat for optimal well-being.

What to Eat and What Not to Eat:

- Eat as per your dosha and use dosha-appropriate spices for cooking your meals.
- Eat a variety of foods of all colors and from all six taste categories. The six taste categories are sweet, sour, salty, pungent, bitter, and astringent.
- Eat foods that grow on plants, not those made in plants.
- Eat "superfoods" that are power-packed with nutrients, fiber, antioxidants, bioflavonoids.
- Eat warm meals that are light and easy to digest.
- Eat foods that are organic, non-GMO, and grown locally.
- Eat a seasonal variety.
- Consume whole grains, leafy greens, fresh fruits, healthy oils, and fats.
- Consume fiber and probiotics.
- Say no to sugar, excess salt, artificial colors, preservatives, food made in factories, white flour, and processed foods. The more the shelf life, the less our life.
- Avoid frequent consumption of ice-cold foods and beverages, especially if you have excess vata or kapha or have vata or kapha dosha predominance. It dilutes our digestive acid and numbs our taste buds.

As you read earlier, I advise you to consume lots of "superfoods" in your diet. So, you might wonder, what are superfoods? Ancient Ayurvedic scriptures have categorized food into three categories: Satvic, Rajasic, and Tamsic. Satvic foods are pure, balanced, offer feelings of calmness, mental clarity, and focus; Rajasic foods are highly stimulating, while Tamsic foods are believed to increase laziness and lethargy. Some also categorize them as foods with positive pranic value, neutral pranic value, and negative pranic value. Depending on your dosha, you can include Satvic and Rajasic foods while eliminating Tamsic food from your diet. The word pranic is derived from the Sanskrit term *Prana* which means the vital life force. Pranic diet includes the pranic foods that categorize foods based on how they affect your lifegiving vital energy or prana.

The word pranic is derived from the Sanskrit term Prana which means the vital life force. Pranic diet includes the pranic foods that categorize foods based on how they affect your lifegiving vital energy or prana.

To make it easy for my global readers, we shall call them superfoods in this book. Superfoods are very similar to pranic foods. These are foods packed with healing life energy. For example, when you plant an apple seed, it will eventually grow into an apple tree under favorable conditions. These are foods packed with nutrients and full of life energy, or prana. They are nutritional powerhouses packed with phytonutrients and antioxidants. They are all-natural, organic, non-GMO, and mostly plant-based. They have unique healing properties and health benefits. They provide a substantial amount of nutrients to nourish your mind, body, and soul.

Here are a few qualities of superfoods:

- Plant-based, made in nature.
- They are organic and non-GMO.
- They are nutritionally dense, power-packed with nutrients, antioxidants, phytochemicals, and soluble, as well as insoluble, fiber.
- They are locally grown and produced.
- They have greater bioavailability.
- Most of them have healing properties and are anti-inflammatory.
- They include a seasonal variety.
- They are lively, vibrant, full of life energy or prana. This means, when you plant them, they will grow into a new plant. For example, when you plant whole grains or legumes, they sprout and develop into a new plant. I do not eat meat because, for example, a chicken breast does not have life energy. It will not reproduce a chicken. For me, it is a dead body, and a dead body cannot give life energy. Yes, it can give you protein, but not life energy.
- Easy to digest and metabolize so that we can absorb the nutrients.

Now that we know the qualities of superfoods, here is the list of some superfoods and why they are considered superfoods:

- Whole grains, like quinoa, barley, brown rice, wild rice, oats, and amaranth: These are packed with nutrients, including protein, fiber, B vitamins, antioxidants, and trace minerals (iron, zinc, copper, and magnesium).
- Mixed beans and legumes like moong beans, black beans,

kidney beans, pinto beans, lima beans, black-eyed beans: These contain protein and fiber. Beans are rich sources of protein, iron, folate, and amino acids.

- Sprouts: Sprouts have very high nutrient levels and are low in calories. They are richer in protein, folate, magnesium, phosphorus, manganese, and vitamins C and K than un-sprouted versions.
- Leafy greens and vegetables like spinach, amaranth greens, dandelion greens, chard, kale, cilantro, collard greens, parsley, fenugreek leaves, mustard greens, arugula, and microgreens: Greens are low in calories, high in nutrients, vitamins, minerals, phytonutrients, and fiber. Most of them are slightly diuretic and help in removing toxins and excess water.
- Cruciferous vegetables like cabbage, cauliflower, broccoli, kale, Brussels sprouts: Rich in nutrients, high in fiber, low in calories.
- Healthy fats like extra virgin olive oil, avocado oil, sesame oil, ghee, tree nuts, like almonds, pistachios, and walnuts; and seeds, like chia seeds, flax seeds, sunflower seeds, and pumpkin seeds: These are all rich in omega-3 fatty acids, protein, vitamin E, and magnesium.
- Fruits like blueberries, blackberries, raspberries, strawberries, mango, kiwi, papaya, apple, bananas, dark grapes, pomegranate, and pineapple: Low in calories, loaded with antioxidants and phytonutrients, high in fiber.
- Root vegetables like sweet potatoes, radishes, and carrots: Rich in soluble and insoluble fiber, which helps to boost the health of gut bacteria.
- Colorful vegetables like tomatoes; eggplant; red, yellow, and orange peppers; artichoke; bok choy; bottle gourd; squash; snake gourd; and zucchini: Rich in phytochemicals and micronutrients.

- Spices like turmeric, ginger, garlic, black pepper, cumin, red chili, paprika, cinnamon, cardamom, fenugreek seeds, mustard seeds, cloves, bay leaves, and cocoa: With powerful antioxidants, they improve immunity, improve digestion, reduce inflammation, and improve metabolism.
- Sweeteners in limited quantities like honey, dates, and jaggery: Honey is anti-inflammatory and has antibacterial properties, dates are high in fiber and antioxidants, while jaggery is rich in magnesium, copper, and iron.

Now we know what superfoods are, let us also understand more about phytonutrients. Plants contain thousands of natural chemicals that help them to flourish and thrive against infections and harmful environmental factors. These life-enhancing organic compounds are called phytonutrients. Phytonutrients are found in nuts, whole grains, fruits, and vegetables. When consumed correctly, they provide us with optimal joint, eye, heart, bone, immune, and brain health.

Phytonutrients act as antioxidants and help our bodies fight free radicals. Free radicals are harmful to our bodies and are generated at the cellular level from everyday activities like stress, lack of sleep, poor diet, pollution, smoking, too much exposure to the sun, too much exercise, lack of proper nutrition, pesticides, chemicals, and processed foods. Studies have proven that the average human being does not consume enough phytonutrients due to their unhealthy dietary habits. To increase phytonutrients in your diet, eat fruits and vegetables of all colors. Nourish your body with a wholesome plant-based diet, including whole grains, nuts, beans, legumes, peas, lentils, leafy green vegetables, and fruits. You are what you eat. The food you eat can either nourish you, or it can put money in your doctor's pocket. Choose wisely.

The Six Tastes of Ayurveda:

We learned about Ayurveda and the importance of digestive fire to attain optimal well-being in earlier chapters. As we saw earlier, according to Ayurveda, there are six different types of tastes, and they are our GPS to optimal health. To determine the right Ayurvedic diet for your body type, we first must determine your dosha, prakriti, and vikriti. You can find an authentic quiz by searching online or visiting https://chopra.com/dosha-quiz to determine your body type and the right diet for your body type. Alternatively, you can schedule an appointment on https://www.krutithakore.com to determine your body type and the right diet for your body type.

We need to know that when we consume all the six tastes in our meals, we are taking a balanced diet. As per Ayurveda, all food is categorized into the above-mentioned six tastes as follows:

The sweet taste comes from foods rich in carbohydrates, proteins, and fat. For example, whole grains, fruits, dairy, nuts, cereals, pasta, bread, oil, honey, maple syrup, and sugar. Sweet taste, when consumed from the right sources, like whole grains, organic food, polyunsaturated and monounsaturated fats, helps calm nerves and build tissues. At the same time, it increases kapha and helps to pacify vata and pitta.

The sour taste comes from foods that have acid, like citric acid, ascorbic acid, lactic acid, acetic acid, etc. A regular dose of sour taste improves your digestive fire, slows down gastric dumping and insulin resistance. But, at the same time, sour taste from some sources is better than others and should not be taken in excess. Try to stick to sources like berries, lemon, and other citrus fruits, yogurt, fermented condiments, etc. Also, this taste increases kapha and pitta. It helps to pacify vata.

The salty taste comes from table salt, fish, soy salt, seaweeds, etc. In the right amount, it helps to improve the taste of food, improves digestion and lubrication, but too much salt can contribute to high blood pressure, water retention, and osteoporosis. Salty taste helps pacify vata but increases pitta and kapha.

The pungent taste is often described as hot and spicy. It comes from peppers, ginger, onions, garlic, mustard, clove, cardamom, cinnamon, chive, leeks, radish, black pepper, etc. These foods are natural antioxidants. They help improve digestion and neutralize cancer-causing free radicals. So, go ahead and add some spice to your food, as well as your life. This food group helps to pacify kapha but increases pitta and vata.

The bitter taste comes from green and yellow vegetables, like eggplant, zucchini, broccoli, cauliflower, cabbage, bitter melon, fenugreek, spinach, kale, almonds with skins, bitter melon, collard greens etc. This group is very high in flavonoids and phytonutrients. It helps to prevent cancer, diabetes, and heart diseases. This food group pacifies kapha and pitta but increases vata.

The astringent taste comes from foods like legumes, beans, tart apple, lemons, cucumbers, figs, cranberries, buttermilk, cherries, celery, bell peppers, potatoes, black tea, green tea, black coffee, dark chocolate, whole wheat, peas, and rye. This regulates digestion and promotes wound healing. This taste pacifies kapha and pitta but increases vata.

So, all these six tastes are the foundation of the Ayurvedic diet. Ayurveda recommends that we consume fresh, cooked meals and not eat stale meals. Also, it recommends eating a plant-based, wholesome diet.

In addition to nurturing your body with the right diet, it is vital to nurture your mind and spirit with the right mental diet for emotional well-being. Hence, form a habit of practicing self-love, meditation, exercise, yoga, mindfulness, laughter, and spending time in nature.

When To Eat:

Eat as per your body's natural rhythms (circadian rhythm). Breakfast should be light. It is important to listen to your body. If you are not very hungry, you may skip breakfast or just have fruit. Lunch can be heavy, but, again, eat a balanced meal. Your plate should contain leafy green vegetables; a small amount of healthy fats; a healthy protein, like legumes or beans; and very few complex carbohydrates, which are a mix of disaccharides and polysaccharides, from whole grains. You would have experienced that when you eat too many simple carbs with lunch, you feel sluggish after lunch due to the sugar rush.

Also, as we saw in part I, Chapter 7, whenever you consume carbohydrates, it converts to sugar, and if that sugar is not utilized, it will be stored as fat by your fat cells. Hence, it is essential to go for a gentle stroll for 15–20 minutes or so after your meals, as that extra movement will help you burn off some sugar and aid digestion. You must keep in mind that strength training enables your body to become more efficient at transporting glucose from your bloodstream to your muscles; hence, it is a great way to prevent or manage prediabetes, diabetes, insulin resistance, and obesity.

Here are some additional tips:

- Stick to three meals per day: breakfast, lunch, and dinner.
- Lunch should be your heaviest meal, and dinner should be very light.
- Maintain daily routine, as far as meals times are concerned.
- Eat dinner at least four hours before your bedtime.
- Don't eat when angry, upset, distracted, or stressed. This is when your sympathetic nervous system is activated, you are in fight or flight mode, and your digestion is very sluggish.
- Wait until one meal is fully digested before eating the next.
- Sit quietly for a few minutes after finishing your meal. Focus

your attention on the sensations in your body, and then take a short walk.

- Avoid snacking between meals.

How To Eat:

It is important to learn the art of eating and understand the science behind it. As we learned in Chapter 6, when you are emotionally disturbed, in a rush, on the go, your sympathetic nervous system is active. The sympathetic nervous system prepares your body for fight or flight. When the sympathetic nervous system is active, blood rushes to larger muscle groups, like legs and arms, and digestion is weak. If you eat when your digestion is weak, your body will produce ama (toxins) instead of producing ojas (vital energy). Now, when you are calm and not distracted by other activities, your parasympathetic nervous system is active, and this is when your digestion is strong, your breathing is slow, and you can think right. Hence, chances are you will make better diet choices when you are calm and digest your food well, which will produce vitality. When your parasympathetic nervous system is active, your body secretes several digestive hormones and enzymes for optimal digestion. Hence you mustn't eat when you are emotionally disturbed, stressed, or distracted by technology.

Here are some tips on how to eat in the right manner:

- Practice mindful eating and chew your food properly, as digestion begins in the mouth.
- Don't use technology or watch movies or TV while eating. While having your meals, focus on the meal, and enjoy your meal. If you have a habit of eating while attending meetings or watching TV, chances are you will overeat because you are not being mindful about what you're eating or how much

you're eating.

- Eat in a quiet, settled, comfortable environment.
- Don't wait till you are starving, because, when you are starving, you will eat whatever you have in front of you. Instead, do proper meal prep. Plan your meals. Make sure that you have all the required ingredients to cook a nutritious meal. Stock up your pantry with superfoods and remove all the processed food/junk food from your pantry, as well as the refrigerator.
- Beware of hidden sugars in your food. Educate yourself and learn to read nutrition labels because sugar can sneak into your food in different ways.
- At the same time, don't overstuff yourself. Research shows that people from the Okinawa region of Japan are one of the healthiest people in the world, and that is because of their diet habits. Not only do they focus on a rich, nutritious diet, they also are very mindful about how much they eat. "Hara Hachi bu" is a commonly followed practice in Japan. It is a Confucian teaching that instructs people to eat until they are 80 percent full or until their belly is eight parts full. This practice facilitates optimal digestion. Every meal does not have to be Thanksgiving dinner, where you have overstuffed yourself so much that you can't even move. Just imagine what happens to your clothes if you overstuff the washing machine. There is no room for the water and detergent to do their job effectively. Similarly, when you overstuff your gut with food, there is no room for digestive juices to freely assimilate with the food and or do their job effectively.
- Always sit down to eat.
- Practice gratitude and bless your food before you eat.
- Take your time. Eat at a pace that allows you to savor your meals and lets your body know when you've eaten enough.

Intermittent Fasting:

This chapter would not be complete without the discussion of intermittent fasting (IF). What is IF? Intermittent fasting means voluntary fasting over a given period. Methods of intermittent fasting include alternate-day fasting, periodic fasting, and daily time-restricted fasting. The most popular method of IF is fasting for 16 hours and eating all your meals within an eight-hour window and is also referred to as "16:8 IF." Other options are 20 hours fasting, then eating meals within a four-hour window, or alternate day fasting (fasting every other day). It takes time to build the habit of intermittent fasting, so you may wish to start with a 12:12 ratio, including no snacking between meals.

There are several benefits of IF, and, in my opinion, the most important benefit is that it teaches "sanyam," which means self-restraint and self-discipline, which is very much needed for optimal well-being.

As I mentioned earlier, the Sanskrit phrase in Ayurvedic texts "langhanam param aushadham" means fasting is the best medicine. This has been supported now by scientific research as well. There are several benefits of IF, and, in my opinion, the most important benefit is that it teaches "sanyam," which means self-restraint and self-discipline, which is very much needed for optimal well-being.

Here is the list of potential benefits of intermittent fasting:

- While overeating and eating when not hungry harm your digestive fire and produces toxins, which leads to chronic inflammation and lifestyle-related illnesses, fasting improves your digestive fire and reduces chronic inflammation.

- Intermittent fasting is an efficient method to remove accumulated toxins and cleanse the body.
- Intermittent fasting balances all the doshas and helps you transition from dis-ease to ease.
- Reduces insulin resistance and leptin resistance.
- Reduces insulin levels in the body and increases levels of HGH, promoting significant weight loss, fat loss, and gain in muscle mass.
- Promotes cellular repair and rejuvenation by removing toxins through a process called autophagy.
- Improves sleep quality, promotes longevity, and improves immunity.
- Improves brain function, concentration, and learning by reducing oxidative stress and inflammation.
- Reduces sluggishness and increases energy levels while restoring vitality.
- Treats lifestyle-related conditions and illnesses like diabetes, hypertension, migraines, obesity.
- Improves skin clarity, resulting in a radiant and youthful appearance by removing toxins from the body.
- Reduces visceral fat (abdominal fat). Abdominal fat is directly related to diabetes, hypertension, and coronary artery disease.
- It may help you prevent diseases like cancer and Alzheimer's.

In short, IF will improve your optimal well-being and the quality of your life.

References:

- *Chopra, D. D., Kshirsagar, D. S., Simon, D. D., Patel, D. S., Porter, D. V., Saint, D. M., Gabriel, R., Stern, E., & Nadarajah, M. (2019, November). The perfect health ayurvedic lifestyle online enrichment program. Session 1 - 15.*

- *Group, E. W. (n.d.). Dirty Dozen™ Fruits and Vegetables with the Most Pesticides. EWG's 2021 Shopper's Guide to Pesticides in Produce | Dirty Dozen. https://www.ewg.org/foodnews/dirty-dozen.php.*

- *Nelson JB. Mindful Eating: The Art of Presence While You Eat. Diabetes Spectr. 2017 Aug;30(3):171-174. doi: 10.2337/ds17-0015. PMID: 28848310; PMCID: PMC5556586. https://www.ncbi.nlm.nih.gov/pmc/articles/PMC5556586/*

- *Van den Driessche JJ, Plat J, Mensink RP. Effects of superfoods on risk factors of metabolic syndrome: a systematic review of human intervention trials. Food Funct. 2018 Apr 25;9(4):1944-1966. doi: 10.1039/C7FO01792H. PMID: 29557436. https://pubmed.ncbi.nlm.nih.gov/29557436/*

- *Waheed Janabi, A. H., Kamboh, A. A., Saeed, M., Xiaoyu, L., BiBi, J., Majeed, F., Naveed, M., Mughal, M. J., Korejo, N. A., Kamboh, R., Alagawany, M., & Lv, H. (2020). Flavonoid-rich foods (FRF): A promising nutraceutical approach against lifespan-shortening diseases. Iranian journal of basic medical sciences, 23(2), 140–153. https://www.ncbi.nlm.nih.gov/pmc/articles/PMC7211351/*

CHAPTER 22

Step 4: Exercise

"Exercise equals endorphins.
Endorphins equals happiness."

We all know that a sedentary lifestyle is one of the major factors in health-related issues, along with unhealthy diet habits and stress. Research shows that "sitting is the new smoking." Today's lifestyle is both a blessing and a curse to humans. Our lives have become easier with the help of machines, but, at the same time, we have invited lifestyle-related illnesses because of our addiction to the remote control and couch. We have become physically inactive, and, hence, we are now more prone to illnesses or conditions like high blood pressure, obesity, diabetes, and high cholesterol.

The temptation to eat junk, unhealthy, processed foods has also increased due to the continuous bombardment of advertisements on television; at the same time, physical activity has decreased.

Unhealthy eating habits, combined with a lack of physical exercise, and an overly stressed and stimulated mind, is a fertile ground for lifestyle-related illnesses. The irony is that our brains are constantly stimulated by electronics and rarely get any rest, while our bodies are continually resting and never getting exercise.

A body in motion stays in motion. Physical exercise has several benefits. It reduces stress, improves sleep, boosts mood, strengthens and tones muscles, promotes a healthy immune system, improves metabolism and digestion, reduces obesity, balances blood sugar, reduces blood pressure and cholesterol, improves brain function, improves cardiovascular health, balances hormones, improves our ability to focus, improves cognitive functions, and increases resting metabolic rate. Also, when your body is tired, your sleep will improve. In short, it facilitates wellness and keeps your body in optimal condition.

Also, both mindful movement and exercise are equally important. One will not replace another. Exercise is a planned activity that either boosts your heart rate through cardio or strengthens your muscles through strength training or both. Mindful movement is intentionally getting up every hour and keeping your body moving. We will review this in our next chapter.

The secret to moving is to start working out and never stop. Keep on moving. Once you start and make it a habit, you would never want to stop because of the benefits you will experience.

The secret to moving is to start working out and never stop. Keep on moving. Once you start and make it a habit, you would never want to stop because of the benefits you will experience. Don't let sedentary distractions prevent you from moving. Use muscles instead of machines to perform physical tasks. Play outdoor games with children and spend quality time with them instead of letting them spend more time on electronic devices. Use a smartwatch or apps on your smartphone to motivate you. Set a goal of completing 10,000 steps in a day, completing 60 minutes of High-Intensity Interval Training (HIIT), or going for hot yoga or a swim or workout class at your local gym.

Ideally, a person should exercise 30 to 45 minutes of exercise per day, five times a week, and it should include cardiorespiratory endurance and strength training. Cardiorespiratory endurance will improve oxygen uptake in the lungs and heart, making them stronger, and strength training protects bone and muscle mass. Any activity which raises your heart rate into the range of 60 to 85 percent of your maximum heart rate (MHR) for at least 15 to 20 minutes of workout time and ideally for 35 to 45 minutes would be considered as exercise. Your MHR is calculated by subtracting your age from 220. Several apps or online calculators are available to calculate your ideal targeted heart rate during exercise. Over and above your age, several factors can determine MHR. You can take help from your trainer, or you may visit www.cdc.gov to determine your MHR. Also, be very mindful and listen to your body. If you experience fatigue or breathlessness, reevaluate your exercise regime. I would also recommend that you talk to your doctor and take their consent before starting a vigorous exercise program.

This does not mean that you need to exercise to the point of exhaustion or to work out for three to four hours a day. As per Ayurveda, exercise is supposed to energize you, make you feel refreshed, and prepare you for the next activity. As everyone is unique, it is essential to identify the right type of exercise that will suit your body type—the one you will benefit the most as per your dosha.

As we read in earlier chapters in Part I, according to Ayurveda, there are three main dosha types: vata, pitta, and kapha.

Vata types are naturally energetic and hyperactive. They are like grasshoppers or hummingbirds. They can hardly sit still, but, at the same time, they get tired easily. They love heavy cardio, which will pump up their heart rate, but this can cause more vata imbalance. If they over-exercise, they will get cramps, feel dizzy, and exhausted. Vata-type people will benefit from grounding exercises like walking, short hikes, tai chi, restorative yoga, light bicycling, strength building, and toning with light or medium weights. These activities will help them stay grounded and develop strength, balance, and tone. They must find indoor workout activities in winter because cold and dry weather will imbalance the vata.

Pitta types are intense and focused. They are natural athletes. They love to compete and love to win. They are naturally strong and agile. They have good stamina and love to work their muscles. They love boxing, boot camps, HIIT, etc., but they need to be careful because they may easily get injured. Also, due to their competitive nature, they can get stressed easily and become out of balance. People with pitta imbalance will benefit the most from swimming, jogging, brisk walks, skiing, biking, outdoor activities, Pilates, and yin yoga. They should make sure to take breaks and keep two days a week for rest. Use meditation, abhyanga (self-massage), and other calming activities to stay calm and grounded.

Kapha types are strong. They have a steady flow of energy and great physical strength. They would excel at endurance sports or any aerobic activities, but they hate to work out. They are more sedentary by nature and getting up to exercise might feel like torture to them. At the same time, once they start the exercise, they enjoy the workout, because it stimulates their mind and body. Sweat is the best medicine for kapha types. Kaphas naturally store fat, and sweat is the natural enemy to their fat. Any exercise that will help them sweat will clear kapha congestion and sluggishness. They would benefit significantly from brisk walking, Zumba, dancing, running, rowing, HIIT, kickboxing, cardio, hot yoga, weight training, or barre class. Aerobic activities that will increase the heart rate are more beneficial for kapha types, and, at the same time, just strength training will not help them much.

All these three body types can benefit from yoga, as there are many different types of yoga, from gentle, restorative, and grounding, to vigorous and sweaty. Nowadays, chair yoga and water yoga practices are also available for people with physical challenges.

What is Yoga?

Yoga is not just a physical exercise; it is also a form of mindful movement, which improves physical, emotional, and spiritual well-being by bringing harmony between mind and body. It is both an art and a science. It is an exercise for both the mind and the body. A set of poses (called asanas), combined with specific breathing techniques (called pranayama), and meditation are the building blocks of yoga. As mentioned above, there are different types of yoga practices to choose from, depending on your dosha type.

The benefits of regular yoga practice are numerous. Yoga improves overall posture, improves joint health, strengthens bones, tones muscles, improves back pain, improves balance, strengthens the spine, reduces stress, calms the mind, improves sleep, improves digestion, improves mood, decreases anxiety, and can benefit those who have PTSD.

Other Forms of Exercise:

In addition to yoga, walking is another form of exercise that anyone can pursue, even without special training. Walking for 30 to 45 minutes a day has several benefits. Walking is excellent for heart health. Some people prefer jogging over brisk walking, which is also good if it works for you, but I favor brisk walking because of its low impact on joints.

If the weather permits, you can walk outside in a park or on the streets. If the weather does not permit, you can walk indoors or do "spot walking or walking in place." You can walk up and down the stairs as well. Any form of walking is good for your heart. Walking also strengthens joints and muscles. Walking does not require any special training, nor does it require a gym. You don't even need special attire. You can go out for a walk at any time of the day, as long as you are walking in a safe neighborhood and the weather is good. Brisk walking improves circulation, strengthens muscles and bones, improves joint flexibility, boosts mood, strengthens the heart, and improves cardiovascular health.

Another of my favorite forms of exercise is swimming. This chapter would have been incomplete without talking about the benefits of swimming. As a former state-level swimmer, I love swimming, but, unlike walking, swimming requires special attire, access to a pool, and some training. Swimming is an excellent form of exercise, as it is a full-body workout that uses all the major muscles of your body. It is the best form of cardio because it increases the heart rate without significant impact or stress on your joints. It builds endurance, muscle strength, cardiovascular health and improves lung capacity. It tones muscles and builds strength. Like yoga and walking, swimming improves

Swimming is an excellent form of exercise, as it is a full-body workout that uses all the major muscles of your body. It is the best form of cardio because it increases the heart rate without significant impact or stress on your joints.

coordination, flexibility, balance, and strength. It reduces stress and is equally as relaxing as walking and yoga.

You may have noticed that I did not discuss another significant benefit of exercise: weight loss. I feel that it is more important to stay healthy and feel good than just lose weight. Weight loss is a secondary benefit, but the most important advantage of exercise is staying healthy and fit. It doesn't matter what form of exercise you pick, as long as you exercise 30 to 45 minutes a day, at least four to five days a week. Start slow, stay steady, and build up the pace if you are new to this.

You may have observed that, no matter how strong-willed a person you are, it is sometimes difficult to discipline yourself to exercise regularly. So, I want to give some tips on how you can incorporate exercise into your daily routine, no matter how busy you are. I will be talking about SMART goals later in the book and how you can use them in any area of your life, like setting exercise goals, eating healthy, exercising, finances, personal development, professional development, etc.

Before I dive into the tips, I want to strongly recommend that you consult with your doctor if you have any health conditions or injuries before starting to exercise. Also, start slowly and increase the intensity if you are new to exercise so that your body gets used to it. Your exercise plans must incorporate a proper warm-up, stretching, and cool-down routine. If you plan to lift weights, start small, and get help from professionals to learn proper techniques to avoid an injury.

Here are a few tips on how to incorporate exercise into your busy schedule:

- If you don't have 30 to 45 minutes at one stretch, exercise 15 to 20 in the morning and 15 to 20 minutes in the evening. When I started, I decided to wake up 30 minutes early to get my daily exercise in.

- It is easy to get bored with exercise and procrastinate because we don't see immediate results. So, keep your eye on the prize. Identify your "why." Your health is important, so always remember that you are doing this for better health or to improve the quality of your life.
- Develop self-love. A person who has developed this quality will never compromise on healthy habits.
- Bring variety into your exercise routine. We might get bored due to a lack of variety. Hence, be open to trying out different activities. This way, you will also ensure that your body does not get used to the same routine. Different types of exercises, like swimming, Zumba, high-intensity interval training (HIIT), strength training, cardio, yoga, jogging, and brisk walking, can be incorporated into your routine.
- Exercise as per your dosha type to get maximum benefit.
- You don't need an expensive gym membership or expensive exercise gear or machines to start exercising. You can buy a few weights and begin at home. There are various YouTube videos on techniques.
- Set up a reward system for yourself. For example, "Once I achieve my exercise goal, I will do my favorite activity." Just keep in mind the reward should not be indulging in junk food or in any habit which will nullify the effect of the exercise.
- Find an accountability partner or exercise buddy.

These were just some tips on how to incorporate exercise into your busy schedule. Start small, keep it simple, stay consistent. Once the habit is formed, it will become easy to keep it up.

References:

- *Saeed SA, Cunningham K, Bloch RM. Depression and Anxiety Disorders: Benefits of Exercise, Yoga, and Meditation. Am Fam Physician. 2019 May 15;99(10):620–627. PMID: 31083878. Available from: https://pubmed.ncbi.nlm.nih.gov/28599839/*
- *Mohammad A, Thakur P, Kumar R, Kaur S, Saini RV, Saini AK. Biological markers for the effects of yoga as complementary and alternative medicine. J Complement Integr Med. 2019 Feb 7;16(1). doi: 10.1515/jcim-2018-0094. PMID: 30735481. Available from: https://pubmed.ncbi.nlm.nih.gov/30735481/*
- *Chopra, D. D., Kshirsagar, D. S., Simon, D. D., Patel, D. S., Porter, D. V., Saint, D. M., Gabriel, R., Stern, E., & Nadarajah, M. (2019, November). The perfect health ayurvedic lifestyle online enrichment program. Session 1–15.*
- *Gupta, S. S., & Sawane, M. V. (2012). A comparative study of the effects of yoga and swimming on pulmonary functions in sedentary subjects. International journal of yoga, 5(2), 128–133. https://www.ncbi.nlm.nih.gov/pmc/articles/PMC3410192/*

CHAPTER 23

Step 5:
Mindful Movement

*"Take time to move; your body longs
to feel alive." - Unknown*

In the previous chapter, we learned about the benefits of exercise, types of exercise for different body types, along with some tips on incorporating exercise into a busy schedule and setting SMART goals. S.M.A.R.T goals are specific, measurable, attainable, relevant or realistic, and time-bound. We shall learn more about SMART goals and how to set them in Chapter 32. Now, you should know that both mindful movement and exercise are equally important. One will not replace another. Mindful movement is about getting up every hour and keeping your body moving. Taking breaks from constant sitting to move your joints will improve joint flexibility. It is important to move throughout the day. Just standing using a standing desk is not enough. The actual movement is needed.

There is a term in the scientific community called "the sitting disease," which refers to metabolic syndrome and the ill effects of an overly sedentary lifestyle. Sitting for a long period increases your risk of chronic health problems like heart disease, diabetes, high blood pressure, varicose veins, urinary tract infections, deep leg thrombosis, obesity, and some cancers. It also weakens your leg, hip, and calf muscles. Immobility for longer periods stops blood circulation, resulting in ankle swelling, painful legs, varicose veins, restless leg syndrome, and even deep vein thrombosis. When you are immobile for long periods (sitting in an airplane, car seat, or chair for hours), your calf muscles are not contracting much, and the blood stagnates.

There is a term in the scientific community called "the sitting disease," which refers to metabolic syndrome and the ill effects of an overly sedentary lifestyle.

Here are a few tips on how you can stay active throughout the day by incorporating a few fun-filled habits:

- Do household chores as a couple or family. Sometimes, household chores are boring, but we can put on some music while working to make the work livelier. An advantage is that doing household chores together strengthens the bond between family members.
- Instead of sitting and talking on the phone, stand up and stroll while talking on the phone.
- Invest in a smartwatch or fitness tracker to monitor your steps and exercise. Set a steps goal. Start small and gradually increase it to 10,000 steps per day. It will also remind you to stand up

and take a few steps if you have been sitting for long. Benefit: If someone tells us to get up and stay active, we feel they are nagging us, but when a smartwatch sends reminders, we won't feel offended. Thus, smartwatches save relationships. Jokes aside, I assure you that this investment is worth the money, as you can track your activity, steps, and exercises. A few of them even remind you to take a break and perform guided breathing exercises to reduce stress.

- If you have a desk job, get a standing workstation so that you have the option of occasionally standing as you work.
- Incorporate outdoor activities with family and kids if the weather permits (going for a stroll together, playing outdoor games, and gardening, for example).
- Put on some music and dance like no one is watching (I assure you that this is fun).
- Take a lunch break away from your desk and go for a short walk after lunch.
- Take the stairs instead of the elevator or escalator.
- Cook some healthy meals together as a family. This strengthens the bond between family members also.
- If you observe yourself sitting for too long, just get up and climb some stairs once or twice.
- When you go shopping, intentionally park your car a greater distance from the entrance of the shop or mall so that you can get a few extra steps toward your daily activity goal. Consider all this fun, and always keep the end in mind. When you feel lazy, remind yourself of the benefits of staying active. In short, keep moving.

I encourage you to be creative and come up with some ideas of your own to keep moving.

References:

- *Baddeley, B., Sornalingam, S., & Cooper, M. (2016). Sitting is the new smoking: where do we stand? The British journal of general practice: the journal of the Royal College of General Practitioners, 66(646), 258. Available from: https://www.ncbi.nlm.nih.gov/pmc/articles/PMC4838429/*
- *Clark, D., Schumann, F., & Mostofsky, S. H. (2015). Mindful movement and skilled attention. Frontiers in human neuroscience, 9, 297. https://www.ncbi.nlm.nih.gov/pmc/articles/PMC4484342/*
- *Chopra, D. D., Kshirsagar, D. S., Simon, D. D., Patel, D. S., Porter, D. V., Saint, D. M., Gabriel, R., Stern, E., & Nadarajah, M. (2019, November). The perfect health ayurvedic lifestyle online enrichment program. Session 1 - 15.*

CHAPTER 24

Step 6: Supplements

᭠᭠᭠

*"All those vitamins aren't to keep death at bay, they're
to keep deterioration at bay." – Jeanne Moreau*

The FDA defines supplements as dietary ingredients taken
by mouth that include vitamins, minerals, amino acids,
antioxidants, phytonutrients, enzyme supplements, herbs
or botanicals, and other substances that can be used to supplement
the diet. They are available in many forms, such as tablets, capsules,
powders, liquids, gummies, and bars.

There is an overabundance of information available on this topic
on the internet and off-net, so it is easy for anyone to get confused.
Some sources say that you don't need supplements if you are eating
right. Others say that no one can eat right, so you need supplements. In
my humble opinion, a typical human being is not an expert on dietary
habits. Nutrients from certain foods are absorbed better by our body
when we eat them raw, while from other foods, nutrients are better

absorbed when we cook them before we consume them. One should not consume any synthetic supplements as our bodies are not designed to metabolize chemicals but supplements that are derived from natural sources are necessary for several reasons. For example, most people do not eat the daily recommended servings of fruits and vegetables.

Day by day, people are getting busier, so cooking two to three times a day is often out of the question. Fresh produce loses nutritional value while it is on the shelf and due to our cooking methods. Adding supplements to your diet will help you meet the nutritional gap in your diet. The problem with most vitamins is that they are synthetic. Also, supplements are not regulated by FDA, so there is a chance that your supplements might not have the nutritional value mentioned on their labels.

Our body generates free radicals due to environmental factors, modern-day lifestyle, stress, and vigorous exercise. Antioxidants assist us in combating these free radicals.

Our body generates free radicals due to environmental factors, modern-day lifestyle, stress, and vigorous exercise. Antioxidants assist us in combating these free radicals. Hence, I believe that adding antioxidants, vitamins, and trace minerals derived from a reliable natural source to the diet, along with eating a healthy, well-balanced diet, proper stress management, and maintaining an active lifestyle by doing moderate to vigorous exercise for 30 to 45 minutes a day four to five times a week will reduce the risk of stroke, heart disease, and all lifestyle as well as age-related illness. All this must be done together.

Along with the vitamins, antioxidants, and trace minerals, I also take a Triphala tablet every day and incorporate herbs into my diet. As a reminder, Triphala is a Sanskrit word for three fruits. It is a powder made up of amalaki (*Phyllanthus emblica*), bibhitaki (*Terminalia bellirica*), and haritaki (*Terminalia chebula*). It helps to detox our digestive system. It is high in antioxidants and has a mild laxative effect. It is also slightly diuretic. For me, it is a gentle way to detox daily. Again, Triphala is not for everyone, so consult an Ayurvedic or health care practitioner before you take it.

We have already learned the importance of micronutrients and vitamins in Chapter 8. In this chapter, I will discuss the benefits of certain supplements like vitamins, minerals, antioxidants, and herbs.

Vitamin A – Vitamin A is a fat-soluble vitamin that supports immune function, vision health, cell growth, cellular reproduction, and cellular communication. It stimulates the production and activity of white blood cells, takes part in remodeling bone, and regulates cell growth and division needed for reproduction.

Vitamin C – Vitamin C, or ascorbic acid, is a water-soluble vitamin. It dissolves in water and is delivered to the body's tissues, but our body does not store it well, so we must take it in daily through food or supplements. It helps control infections and wound healing. It is a powerful antioxidant that can neutralize harmful free radicals. It is needed to make collagen, a fibrous protein in connective tissue woven throughout various systems in the body: nervous, immune, bone, cartilage, blood, and others. Vitamin C helps to make several hormones and chemical messengers used in the brain and nerves.

Vitamin B1 (thiamine) – Thiamine is a water-soluble vitamin that plays a vital role in the growth and function of various cells. It is stored in small amounts in the liver, so a daily intake of thiamine-rich foods is needed.

Vitamin B2 (riboflavin) – Riboflavin is a water-soluble vitamin naturally present in food or taken as a supplement. Our gut bacteria can produce small amounts of riboflavin but not enough to meet dietary needs. Hence, it is important to have a healthy diversity of gut bacteria, as riboflavin is a key component of coenzymes involved with the growth of cells, energy production, and the breakdown of fats, steroids, and medications.

Vitamin B3 (niacin) – This is a water-soluble vitamin that works as a coenzyme, and more than 400 enzymes depend on it for various reactions. Niacin helps convert nutrients into energy, create cholesterol and fats, create and repair DNA, and has antioxidant effects.

Vitamin B5 (pantothenic acid) – Vitamin B5 is a water-soluble vitamin and is used to make coenzyme A (CoA), a chemical compound that helps enzymes to build and break down fatty acids as well as perform other metabolic functions.

Vitamin B6 – Vitamin B6 is a water-soluble vitamin naturally present in many foods, added to others, and available as a dietary supplement. It helps in a wide variety of functions in the body and is highly versatile, with involvement in more than 100 enzyme reactions, primarily concerned with protein metabolism. Also, research shows that it helps to improve cardiovascular health by lowering homocysteine levels. As per research, B6, along with folic acid and B12, may help reduce the chances of heart attack and stroke.

Vitamin B7 (biotin) – Biotin deficiency can lead to hair loss, skin, and nail problems. Biotin plays a vital role in assisting enzymes in breaking down fats, carbohydrates, and proteins in food. It also helps to regulate signals sent by cells and the activity of genes.

Vitamin B9 (folic acid or folate) – Folate is the natural form of vitamin B9, water-soluble, and naturally found in many foods. It helps to form RNA and DNA. It is involved in protein metabolism. It plays a key role in breaking down homocysteine, an amino acid that can exert harmful effects in the body if it is present in high amounts. Folate is also needed to produce healthy red blood cells and is critical during periods of rapid growth, such as during pregnancy and fetal development.

Vitamin B12 – Vitamin B12 is naturally found in animal products, so it is important that vegans and vegetarians supplement themselves with this vitamin. Vitamin B12 is needed to form red blood cells and DNA. It is also a key player in the function and development of brain and nerve cells.

Vitamin D3 – Vitamin D, nicknamed "the sunshine vitamin," is highly important for several body functions. Vitamin D is both a nutrient we eat and a hormone our body makes. It is a fat-soluble vitamin that helps the body absorb and retain calcium and phosphorus, which are important for bone health. Some research shows that it can reduce cancer cell growth, help control infections, and reduce inflammation. It is produced in our skin in the presence of the sun's ultraviolet B (UVB) rays. Most people don't spend enough time in the sun or use sunscreen lotions; hence, they are deficient in this vitamin, and they should take supplements. People with darker skin have melanin, which protects them against absorption of UVB rays, and, hence, they are deficient in vitamin D, even if they spend time in the sun.

Vitamin E – Vitamin E protects from free radicals and supports cellular health. Vitamin E is a fat-soluble vitamin, so you need to consume it with food. Make sure to consult a professional before you use it so that you do not take an overdose of vitamin E.

Vitamin K – Found in leafy green vegetables and fermented foods, this fat-soluble vitamin is easily broken down by our body, so it is difficult to overdose on it, as any excess amount is removed from the body through stool or urine. It helps to make various proteins that are needed for blood clotting and the building of bones.

Calcium – Calcium is a mineral linked with healthy bones and teeth. It also plays an important role in blood clotting, helps muscle contraction, and regulates normal heart rhythms and nerve functions. About 99 percent of the body's calcium is stored in the bones, and the remaining one percent is found in blood, muscle, and other tissues. The body gets the calcium it needs in two ways. One is by eating foods or supplements that contain calcium, and the other is by drawing from calcium in the body. If one does not eat enough calcium-containing foods, the body will remove calcium from the bones resulting in osteoporosis. Osteoporosis is a condition that causes bones to become weak and brittle to the extent that even mild stress can cause a fracture. This is a common condition in the elderly, and your doctor may recommend a bone density test to determine the health of your bones once you reach mid 50's.

Magnesium – Magnesium assists more than 300 enzymes in performing important biological functions. It also plays an important role in regulating blood sugar, blood pressure, muscle, and nerve functions. Magnesium also acts as an electrical conductor that contracts muscles and makes the heartbeat steady.

Zinc – Zinc is required by the body in small amounts but plays a vital role in the creation of DNA, growth of cells, repair, and healing of damaged tissues. It is crucial during pregnancy because it helps cells grow and multiply. It supports the development and functioning of immune cells and, hence, a zinc deficiency can lead to lower immune function.

Manganese – Manganese helps build bones and heal wounds.

Iron – Iron is an essential mineral that helps maintain healthy blood. Iron is a major component of hemoglobin, a protein in red blood cells that carries oxygen from your lungs to all parts of the body. Without enough iron, there aren't enough red blood cells to transport oxygen, causing fatigue.

Sodium – Our body requires a small amount of sodium to conduct nerve impulses, contract and relax muscles, and maintain the proper balance of water and minerals. It is estimated that we need about 500 mg of sodium daily for these vital functions, but due to the consumption of processed food or junk food, we consume too much sodium in the diet, leading to high blood pressure, heart disease, and stroke.

Chromium – Chromium is an essential mineral required by our body in trace amounts. Chromium enhances the action of the hormone insulin and helps in the breakdown and absorption of carbohydrates, proteins, and fats. Vitamins B3 and C help to improve the absorption of chromium.

Selenium – This is an important trace mineral and an essential component of various enzymes and proteins, which are called selenoproteins. These enzymes and proteins help to make DNA and protect against cell damage and infections. They are also involved in the reproduction and the metabolism of thyroid hormones.

Lecithin – Lecithin helps the body more effectively absorb vitamin E. Research indicates that lecithin may help in reducing LDL and increasing HDL. Lecithin supplements show promising results in lowering blood cholesterol levels. It may also help in improving immune function.

Lycopene – Lycopene is a natural compound found in bright red fruits and vegetables, like tomatoes, watermelon, and grapefruit. Lycopene is a carotenoid: yellow, orange, or red pigments, which give these colors to plants. A diet rich in lycopene may protect against stroke and reduce the risk of prostate cancer and other types of cancer.

Lutein – Lutein is also a naturally occurring carotenoid, which is absorbed best when taken with a diet rich in fat. It has anti-inflammatory properties, several benefits in improving eye health, cognitive function, and reducing risks of cancer.

Green tea extract – Natural green tea extract offers phytonutrients to help protect against cell-damaging free radicals.

Ginseng – Ginseng is very popular these days and research through controlled trials shows that this herb has the potential to improve focus, concentration, memory, and boost mood. Research shows that this herb when taken orally can improve your response to environmental stress and overall well-being. As this herb improves focus, concentration, and mental alertness, I recommend not consuming it later in the day as it might impact your sleep. It is safe to consume it for a shorter duration. The most common side effect is insomnia, so this might not be for you if you have trouble sleeping.

Rhodiola Rosea – Rhodiola Rosea extract is a popular dietary supplement among active individuals, including athletes, as it can improve your body's resistance to physical and behavioral stresses for fighting fatigue and depression. Over and above that, recent studies have shown promising results due to its anti-aging, anti-inflammation, immunostimulating, DNA repair, and anti-cancer properties.

Milk thistle – Milk thistle has been used by herbalists for hundreds of years to treat nonalcoholic fatty liver syndrome, hepatitis and to protect the liver from environmental toxins. Research shows that Milk thistle exhibits its hepatoprotective properties by three major mechanisms: 1) serving as an antioxidant, 2) an anti-inflammatory, and 3) an antifibrotic substance.

Dandelion – Research shows that dandelion has several beneficial properties; it is anti-diabetic, anti-oxidative, and anti-inflammatory. It may also help reduce water retention and effectively treat diabetes and obesity. In some studies, dandelion components were shown to inhibit oxidative stress in liver injury, reduce high cholesterol, and reverse streptozotocin-induced diabetes.

CoQ10 – This is a compound made by your body and stored in mitochondria. It helps generate energy in your cells. It is naturally produced by your body, but research shows that the production decreases with age. Hence, it is vital to get CoQ10 through supplementation. Health conditions like heart disease, brain disorders, diabetes, and cancer have been linked to low levels of CoQ10.

Omega-3 fatty acids – These have several benefits, including lowering blood triglyceride levels. High triglyceride levels can increase the chances of heart disease and stroke. They are also anti-inflammatory and may reduce stiffness and joint pain. Some research suggests that omega-3s may help protect against Alzheimer's disease and dementia.

Glucosamine and chondroitin – These supplements have been clinically shown to support joint health.

Triphala – Triphala helps to detox our digestive system. It is high in antioxidants and has a mild laxative effect. It is also slightly diuretic. In addition to that, Triphala has numerous other benefits. It may be used for its antioxidant, anti-inflammatory, immunomodulating, antibacterial, antimutagenic, and hypoglycemic properties. It also has chemoprotective and radioprotective effects. Research shows that the polyphenols in Triphala modulate the human gut microbiome and thereby promote the growth of beneficial *Bifidobacteria* and *Lactobacillus* while inhibiting the growth of undesirable gut microbes. The bioactivity of Triphala is elicited by gut microbiota to generate a variety of anti-inflammatory compounds.

Turmeric – This powerful golden herb is like powdered gold and is used in Indian and Asian cooking. Its active component is curcumin, which is highly anti-inflammatory and a powerful antioxidant. It purifies the blood, improves blood flow, reduces inflammation, improves immunity and joint health. It protects against heart disease, improves respiratory health, loosens mucus, heals wounds, and cures infections. An herb blend of milk thistle, dandelion root, and turmeric supports normal liver metabolic activity and function. It also offers antioxidant protection from free radicals.

This powerful golden herb is like powdered gold and is used in Indian and Asian cooking.

Brahmi – Brahmi has strong anti-inflammatory and adaptogenic properties and improves attention, memory, focus, and mental performance. It can reduce symptoms of ADHD and restlessness.

Bitter melon – An extremely bitter vegetable but has powerful cleansing properties. It balances excess kapha. It is a staple in Asian and Indian cuisine and is packed with nutrients and antioxidants. Research suggests that it may help lower blood sugar levels and promote insulin secretion.

Ashwagandha – This is a potent adaptogen that helps your body manage stress more effectively. Research has shown that it reduces cortisol levels, which is a stress hormone, decreases anxiety, improves sleep, and enhances memory and muscle growth. It improves immunity and reduces inflammation.

This is a potent adaptogen that helps your body manage stress more effectively.

Holy basil or Tulsi – This is an adaptogen with anti-inflammatory properties. It is antiarthritic, anticoagulant, antidiabetic, antimicrobial, and antioxidant. It reduces stress hormones, improves immunity, helps fight colds and flu, loosens mucus, decreases inflammation, improves brain function, improves GI function, stabilizes blood sugar levels, and promotes longevity.

Licorice root – Native to Europe and Asia, licorice root may help reduce inflammation and fight viruses and bacteria. It also appears to offer relief from sore throats and promotes oral health by protecting against dental cavities.

Cardamom – This herb is commonly used in Indian and Asian cooking and is well known for its fragrance. It is called the queen of spices and has been used in Ayurvedic medicine for ages. Research suggests it may help reduce blood pressure levels.

Cumin – Cumin ignites the digestive fire, improves digestion, boosts the activity of digestive enzymes.

Saffron – Saffron is a powerful antioxidant. It is a great mood booster and reduces anxiety and depression, as well as reduces PMS symptoms. Research shows it may also reduce appetite and help with weight loss.

Fennel and fennel seeds – Highly nutritious, fennel and fennel seeds contain powerful antioxidants and potent plant compounds. Studies show that they have anti-inflammatory, anticancer, antioxidant, and antimicrobial properties. People who take a diet rich in fennel and fennel seeds have a lower risk of chronic conditions like heart disease, obesity, cancer, neurological diseases, and type 2 diabetes. They reduce inflammation, reduce appetite, aid in digestion, and have a cooling effect. They, in combination with cumin and coriander, help reduce excess pitta.

Ginger – Ginger is a powerful antioxidant with excellent anti-inflammatory properties. It is also antimicrobial, like turmeric, holy basil, onion, and garlic. It has heating properties that help to ignite the digestive fire, improves digestion, loosens excess mucus, balances excess kapha, helps in respiratory diseases, reduces nausea and vomiting, lowers blood sugar levels, treats chronic indigestion, and reduces cholesterol levels. It may also help with weight loss.

Garlic – Garlic is highly nutritious and low in calories. It is a potent antioxidant and helps to detoxify heavy metals in the body. It is also antimicrobial and anti-inflammatory. It helps reduce colds, flu, and cough symptoms, and it loosens mucus. It helps lower cholesterol, oxidative stress, and blood pressure.

Onion – Although not an herb, I included onions in this section along with lemon due to their medicinal properties. These are packed with antioxidants and are highly anti-inflammatory. They contain 25 different antioxidants. Onions can help reduce inflammation, decrease cholesterol and triglycerides. Reduces risk of heart disease, high blood pressure, cancer, and diabetes.

Lemon – Lemons are an excellent source of vitamin C and soluble fiber.

Chili peppers – Rich in vitamins and minerals, along with other plant compounds, like capsaicin and antioxidant carotenoids. They improve digestive health and metabolism; reduce weight; alleviate migraines; may reduce risks of cancer; fight fungal infections, colds, and the flu; provides joint pain relief; fight inflammation; support cardiovascular health; may improve cognitive functions; and may improve longevity. They have heating properties, helps to reduce excess kapha, and can increase pitta dosha when consumed in excess.

Black pepper – Black pepper is high in antioxidants and has anti-inflammatory properties. It may improve digestion, promote gut health, reduce nausea and vomiting, improve blood sugar levels, and decrease cholesterol levels.

Cinnamon – This spice has antiviral, antibacterial, anti-inflammatory, and antifungal properties. It is packed with antioxidants. It has prebiotic properties that can improve gut health. It may help reduce blood pressure, blood sugar, and decrease the risk of type 2 diabetes. It also relieves digestive discomfort.

Lavender – Lavender has a calming effect. It may help improve sleep, calm your nerves, reduce anxiety. It could help treat skin blemishes. May offer a natural remedy for pain, lower blood pressure and heart rate. It could relieve asthma symptoms. Ease menopausal hot flashes and potentially promotes hair growth.

Chamomile – Highly anti-inflammatory. May lower blood sugar. Helps with sleep and relaxation.

Fenugreek – Rich in fiber and protein, bitter in taste. Helps balance excess kapha. Highly anti-inflammatory, it may help reduce and balance blood sugar levels and LDL cholesterol. Helps in detoxification and appetite control.

Keep in mind that just consuming supplements or just exercising, or just eating healthy, or just meditation will not suffice. Sometimes people think that supplements or vigorous exercise will give them the permission to pursue unhealthy dietary habits, or it gives them the permission to smoke or consume alcohol. This mindset will lead to more harm than the benefits of supplements and exercise.

A reminder due to the dietary habits of most people, they run a greater risk of vitamin and mineral deficiency compared to overdosage. Also, one cannot overdose on water-soluble vitamins because our bodies do not store them well. Hence, we need to take them through a wholesome diet consisting of a wide variety of fruits, vegetables, dairy, whole grains, and healthy fats or add supplements made from natural sources to help you bridge the nutritional gap. However, we must be careful when taking fat-soluble vitamins because any excess amount that is not immediately needed by the body is absorbed and stored in fat tissue or the liver. If too much is stored, it can become toxic. Also, not all herbal supplements are for everyone, so don't consume herbal supplements without consulting a professional or a licensed healthcare provider.

References:

- *U.S. Department of Health and Human Services. (n.d.). Dietary Supplement Fact Sheets. NIH Office of Dietary Supplements. https://ods.od.nih.gov/factsheets/list-all/.*

- Buscemi, S., Corleo, D., Di Pace, F., Petroni, M. L., Satriano, A., & Marchesini, G. (2018). The Effect of Lutein on Eye and Extra-Eye Health. Nutrients, 10(9), 1321. https://www.ncbi.nlm.nih.gov/pmc/articles/PMC6164534/

- U.S. Department of Health and Human Services. (n.d.). Office of dietary supplements - riboflavin. NIH Office of Dietary Supplements. Retrieved December 2, 2021, from https://ods.od.nih.gov/factsheets/Riboflavin-HealthProfessional/.

- Chopra, D. D., Kshirsagar, D. S., Simon, D. D., Patel, D. S., Porter, D. V., Saint, D. M., Gabriel, R., Stern, E., & Nadarajah, M. (2019, November). The perfect health ayurvedic lifestyle online enrichment program. Session 1–15.

- Peterson CT, Denniston K, Chopra D. Therapeutic Uses of Triphala in Ayurvedic Medicine. J Altern Complement Med. 2017 Aug;23(8):607-614. doi: 10.1089/acm.2017.0083. Epub 2017 Jul 11. PMID: 28696777; PMCID: PMC5567597. Available from: https://pubmed.ncbi.nlm.nih.gov/28696777/

- Singh, N., Bhalla, M., de Jager, P., & Gilca, M. (2011). An overview on ashwagandha: a Rasayana (rejuvenator) of Ayurveda. African journal of traditional, complementary, and alternative medicines: AJTCAM, 8(5 Suppl), 208–213. https://www.ncbi.nlm.nih.gov/pmc/articles/PMC3252722/

- Jiang TA. Health Benefits of Culinary Herbs and Spices. J AOAC Int. 2019 Mar 1;102(2):395–411. doi: 10.5740/jaoacint.18-0418. Epub 2019 Jan 16. PMID: 30651162. https://pubmed.ncbi.nlm.nih.gov/30651162/

- Krishnaswamy K. Traditional Indian spices and their health significance. Asia Pac J Clin Nutr. 2008;17 Suppl 1:265–8. PMID: 18296352. https://pubmed.ncbi.nlm.nih.gov/18296352/

- Achufusi TGO, Patel RK. Milk Thistle. [Updated 2021 Sep 15]. In: StatPearls [Internet]. Treasure Island (FL): StatPearls Publishing; 2022 Jan-. Available from: https://www.ncbi.nlm.nih.gov/books/NBK541075/

- *Jin, Y., Cui, R., Zhao, L., Fan, J., & Li, B. (2019). Mechanisms of Panax ginseng action as an antidepressant. Cell proliferation, 52(6), e12696.* *https://www.ncbi.nlm.nih.gov/pmc/articles/PMC6869450/*
- *Li, Y., Pham, V., Bui, M., Song, L., Wu, C., Walia, A., Uchio, E., Smith-Liu, F., & Zi, X. (2017). Rhodiola rosea L.: an herb with anti-stress, anti-aging, and immunostimulating properties for cancer chemoprevention. Current pharmacology reports, 3(6), 384–395.* *https://www.ncbi.nlm.nih.gov/pmc/articles/PMC6208354/* *Wirngo, F. E., Lambert, M. N., & Jeppesen, P. B. (2016). The Physiological Effects of Dandelion (Taraxacum Officinale) in Type 2 Diabetes. The review of diabetic studies: RDS, 13(2-3), 113–131.* *https://doi.org/10.1900/RDS.2016.13.113*

CHAPTER 25

Step 7: Hydration

*"Pure water is the world's first
and foremost medicine."*

The human body is 60 percent water, but many people don't realize that water plays a vital role in bodily functions. Water helps us improve our health, fitness, and appearance. **Here are a few benefits of drinking water:**

- Water regulates body temperature. It is essential to stay hydrated to maintain a normal body temperature. We lose water through perspiration, as it helps us to stay cool, but if we don't replenish lost water, we become dehydrated. Dehydration has serious effects on our body, varying from fatigue to serious consequences like high blood pressure or seizures.
- It helps improve joint health. Water helps us improve joint health by providing lubrication to our joints and tissues.

Optimal joint health helps us to prevent arthritis so that we can enjoy a long, active, pain-free life.

- It regulates digestion and helps with nutrient absorption. Drinking enough water helps our digestive tract to break down food easily. It also aids in dissolving vitamins, minerals, and other nutrients present in our food and in transporting them to our cells.

- Improves blood oxygen circulation. Our body needs water to transfer essential nutrients, as well as oxygen, to different organs, and water plays a vital role in this process.

- Improves focus by helping with brain function. Water helps improve our brain function, focus, alertness, and memory. It also helps us improve our mood.

- It helps reduce body weight by decreasing caloric intake and boosts metabolic rate. At times, our brain mistakes thirst for hunger, and we reach for food when we are thirsty. If we stay hydrated, we can reduce caloric intake. Water helps boost metabolic rate also. A research study has proven that by drinking just 500 mL of water, we can boost our metabolic rate by 30 percent. The metabolic rate is directly proportional to energy expenditure. Increase in energy expenditure results in increased weight loss. Also, as water improves digestion, drinking enough water, along with eating a healthy diet and exercise, can speed up fat loss and weight loss.

- Improves the appearance of skin. Even though water intake alone cannot prevent visible signs of aging on your skin, it does play a key role in keeping our skin well-hydrated and improving collagen production. Also, as we saw above, it helps in efficiently transporting nutrients in our body at the cellular level.

- It helps flush out waste from our body and prevents

constipation. Our body eliminates waste through sweat, urine, and defecation. When we sweat, we lose water, as well as electrolytes. Water also helps our kidneys function at an optimal level, as they are our body's filtration plants, and they remove toxins via urine. When our body efficiently removes toxins, we eliminate the possibility of frequent headaches and migraines. Also, just consuming fiber is not enough for smooth bowel movements. Fiber, along with water, is required so that our body can remove solid wastes through bowel movements. Adding fiber and water to our diet will ensure that we have smooth bowel movements. Thus, it can help us to prevent piles (hemorrhoids) and anal fissures.

- It helps with performance during physical activity and exercise. As we saw earlier, water helps boost metabolic rate. When our metabolic rate is boosted, we feel more energized. Boosts in our energy levels will improve our performance during physical activity and exercise. Also, when we exercise, our body produces free radicals. Free radicals are harmful, so our bodies must remove them efficiently. Water speeds up the removal of free radicals and toxins. When we exercise, our muscles also produce lactic acid, which results in discomfort and soreness. Water speeds up the removal of lactic acid from our muscles so that we can exercise without discomfort and bounce back quickly from soreness.

- It helps heal certain medical conditions, like urinary tract infections, kidney stones, constipation, high blood pressure, diabetes, hemorrhoids and anal fissures, common cold and cough, migraines, and headaches.

- Water prevents dehydration. As water is essential for several bodily functions, lack of enough water causes dehydration. There are severe consequences to our health from dehydration.

Now, we already know the health benefits of water, so the question is, how much water should we drink?

According to the <u>National Academies of Sciences, Engineering, and Medicine</u>, the recommended water intake (from all beverages and foods) is:

- about 15.5 cups (125 ounces) daily for men
- about 11.5 cups (91 ounces) daily for women

According to the National Academies of Sciences, Engineering, and Medicine, the recommended water intake (from all beverages and foods) is:

- *about 15.5 cups (125 ounces) daily for men*
- *about 11.5 cups (91 ounces) daily for women*

Out of this, we likely get around 20 percent of our daily water requirements from the food we eat. For the rest, 80 percent, we should drink enough water.

Those who are into gardening know that different types of plants have different watering requirements. For example, succulents do not need as much water as lotus, and the daisy needs well-drained soil. Similarly, as per Ayurveda, water requirement varies from person to person. Since the primary composition of kapha type people is earth and water, kapha types may not need much water compared to vata and pitta types. Also, kapha and vata types benefit from *warm* water, especially during winter and early spring, or if they experience sinus congestion due to mucous accumulation. Warm water or non-caffeinated herbal ginger lemon tea effectively removes excess kapha and mucus. Pitta types benefit from cold water. Also, during summer, CCF tea can cool down aggravated pitta. CCF tea is made by boiling cumin, coriander and fennel seeds in water. Visit https://www.krutithakore.com/recipes/cumin-coriander-fennel-tea-ccf-tea for the recipe. Excess kapha or mucus is gross and sticky, which is very similar to grease and oil stuck in a pan. Hot or warm water is highly effective in removing grease from the pan; in the same way, warm water or herbal teas, as mentioned above, are very effective in removing built-up kapha or mucus. Virgin hot toddy is perfect for balancing kapha and igniting the sluggish digestive fire. For recipe visit www.krutithakore.com/recipes/virgin-hot-toddy.

Many people do not like the taste of tap water, and they also know that tap water may have harmful heavy metals and contaminants. Hence, they don't drink enough water, or they use bottled water or end up drinking a sugary sports drink, sodas, or fruit juices. They do so without realizing the harmful consequences of microplastics and carcinogens in bottled water, or the sugar, artificial colorings, artificial sweeteners, and preservatives present in a sports drink, fruits juices, and sodas on their health.

Here are a few tips on staying hydrated:

- Drink two glasses of warm water first thing in the morning. Add the juice of one lemon to it. Lemon juice acts as a gentle detoxifying agent.
- Invest in a good quality water purification system at home. Not Brita or PUR or anything similar to those, as they are not true water purifiers. Don't get me wrong, they do remove some impurities, but not all. They just remove *visible* macro-impurities but are not equipped to remove microbial contaminants, toxins, and other soluble impurities. I also don't

recommend bottled water for several reasons, including the harmful effects of plastic on the environment and the presence of microplastics and carcinogens in plastic bottles.

- Infuse your drinking water with fruits and vegetables, like pineapple, strawberries, blueberries, oranges, lemons and limes, cucumbers, mint, etc., to give it some flavor and nutrients while also making it more visually appealing.
- Always carry filtered water from your home in a glass bottle with you. Keep it on your desk while you work. It will remind you to stay hydrated.
- Also, carry filtered water with you when you go out for exercise or while you are involved in any kind of physical activity.

Now that we have learned the importance of drinking water and staying hydrated, the question arises about whether our drinking water is safe enough to consume without treating it at home.

In 2014, the Flint, Michigan, water crisis began, which led all of us to wonder if our drinking water was safe enough to consume. In the case of Flint, it was found out that, due to insufficient water treatment, lead from the water pipes had leaked into the drinking water, and more than 100,000 residents had been exposed to elevated lead levels. The water we consume either comes from surface sources, like lakes, rivers, springs, and reservoirs, or from underground sources, like wells, permeable rocks, or aquifers.

Our drinking water may be contaminated by pharmaceutical waste, harmful organic chemicals from extensive use of pesticides and chemical fertilizers, contaminants from nature, radionuclides, microbial contaminants from sewage, and heavy metal contaminants from the pipes themselves. Practically speaking, no provider can treat millions of gallons of water to make it safe for consumption. Even if the water is completely purified, there is the chance of corrosion and seepage of contaminants into the water due to a decades-old distribution network.

Below is a list of a few contaminants that can be found in our drinking water. To find the impurities in the tap water in your area, visit https://www.ewg.org/tapwater/. These can only be effectively removed by a high-quality water filtration system instead of a simple water filter.

- Lead
- Mercury
- Asbestos
- Benzene
- Radon
- Chlorine
- Aluminum
- Ammonia
- Arsenic
- Nitrate and Nitrites
- Bacteria
- Viruses
- Algae
- Radium
- Uranium
- Selenium
- Copper

Most of these contaminants have a very slow adverse effect on our body, so it might take years for someone to realize the aftereffects. Research shows that these contaminants have been associated with an increased risk of cancer, reproductive problems, and irreversible kidney and liver damage.

For the above-mentioned reasons, people fear that tap water is not safe for consumption and, instead, buy bottled water, feeling that they are taking care of their health. I feel that bottled water quality is no better than tap water. Buying bottled water is a waste of money and harmful to the environment. Often these bottles have been stored out in the sun and heat. When plastic bottles are exposed to heat and sun, they release carcinogens. Also, bottled water has been known to release microplastics, which are harmful to our health. Due to the cost factors, people avoid cooking with bottled water. They use tap water for cooking, and, in this case, what is the point of wasting money by buying bottled water just for drinking? Some people feel that boiling tap water is a better alternative, but, in that case, they are increasing the concentration of heavy metals and chemicals present in water.

So, what is the solution? The best option is to take charge of your drinking water at your home and purify the water which is used for drinking and cooking. Invest in a good quality water purification system that can remove microparticles and not just large particles and contaminants. Either use filtered water, or your body becomes the filter. The second option takes a significant toll on your kidneys and liver at the cost of your health and life. To find a safe alternative to tap or bottled water, contact me by visiting www.krutithakore.com.

References:

- *Centers for Disease Control and Prevention. (2014, April 7). Water-related diseases and contaminants in public water systems. Centers for Disease Control and Prevention. Retrieved December 2, 2021, from https://www.cdc.gov/healthywater/drinking/public/water_diseases.html*
- *The Water in You: Water and the Human Body. (n.d.). https://www.usgs.gov/special-topic/water-science-school/science/water-you-water-and-human-body.*

CHAPTER 26

Step 8:
Healthy Emotions

‑‑‑‑‑

*"Do not dwell in the past, do not dream
of the future, concentrate the mind on
the present moment." — Buddha.*

The purpose of this book is to help you realize that you, as a
human being, are not just your body. Your body and mind
are instruments through which your consciousness (soul)
expresses itself and experiences life. You must remember that your
identity does not depend on your instruments. Just like you have a
mind and a body, you also have other things or instruments, like a
car, a house, a computer, a job, and stuff, but these should not define
you. Your well-being in life depends on you becoming the master
of your instruments and not the other way around. You would never
let your car tell you where to drive, right? In the same manner, the

desires of your body and mind should not control you. You are the master of your body and mind (your instruments).

When your mind is quiet, you will be guided by your intelligence, your consciousness, and higher power so that you can decipher between right and wrong. When we do not master our minds and emotions, our well-being suffers. Our capacity to make the right choices decreases. This leads to becoming a victim to temptations, and in your daily life, you will come across many such temptations. They can be as simple as eating brownies loaded with sugar or becoming a couch potato and binge-watching Netflix to something more severe like spending the money you don't have on things you don't need. These are just a few examples, but there is no shortage of temptations during current times when a majority of us believe in YOLO (You only live once), but the truth is you live every day, and your actions will determine the quality of your life so be mindful of your actions and be the master of your mind and emotions, not a slave. At the same time, we must nurture our minds and body to attain optimal well-being. It is important to nurture our body with the right nutrition and keep it moving. Also, it is important to nurture our minds with the right thoughts, positive experiences, and positive emotions. If we treat our mind and body poorly, it will result in disharmony and disease.

My mentor always used to say, "Life is not a straight line." Life is filled with ups and downs, just like our EKG. Every one of us will have situations and challenges in life. It's not about having a smooth, easy life; it is about how well we respond to these challenges, which

> *When your mind is quiet, you will be guided by your intelligence, your consciousness, and higher power so that you can decipher between right and wrong.*

will determine our optimal well-being. It is a huge relief to realize that our well-being depends on us and how well we respond to any situation in life. Instead of giving control to anyone or anything else, we take our control back. No one is responsible for my state of mind or my emotions except me. If there is a problem, the solution is in the mirror.

This mindset gives us the ability to take control and overcome our victim mentality. People these days have low tolerance and a habit of blaming everything and everyone else for their emotional and mental state. They feel it is natural to get angry or upset if things do not go their way in life.

For example, when I am stuck in a traffic jam, I can choose my response. I can either get angry or stay calm. If I get angry, I let that situation have power over me. I am letting that situation control my emotions, but when I choose to stay calm, listen to some great music, or some positive mental attitude audiobook while I am stuck in traffic, I am in control of my emotions.

We must always remember that we have power over situations in life. When we form a habit of not letting our life situations get the best of our emotions, we develop emotional stability, which helps us, even when more severe situations arise. Developing emotional stability is like developing muscle. The more you exercise it, the stronger it becomes.

Life is never going to be free of stress and resistance. Hence, our physical and emotional health greatly depends on our ability to handle stress. Our ability to develop nurturing relationships also depends on our emotional health. Science has already proven that there is a strong correlation between our physical health and emotional health. Hence, it is very important to learn to develop healthy emotions.

You may have come across two types of people in life. One type is not bothered by anything, while the other type is bothered by everything. One type always finds hope in any situation, while the other feels every situation is like doomsday. You may also have seen that people love to hang around the first category, while they avoid people of the second category. When people of the first category enter any room, the room lights up. They are positive, cheerful, always uplift others, and, in any situation, they remain calm and hopeful. They have this unique ability to stay calm under pressure and respond well to any situation. While in the case of people of the second category, the room lights up when they leave the room. They are negative, complain about everything, are constantly stressed, and worry a lot. Their negativity is contagious, and they drain the energy of everyone around them. They have a habit of making a mountain out of a molehill. They tend to react to every situation and are eager to put people down. Hence, no one likes to hang around them. The reason is very simple. You cannot attract bees with vinegar. Similarly, you cannot be a people magnet with a negative mindset and attitude.

You cannot attract bees with vinegar. Similarly, you cannot be a people magnet with a negative mindset and attitude.

Now there are two types of emotions. Positive or healthy emotions lead to excellent mental and emotional health. Positive emotions increase the level of happy hormones (serotonin, dopamine, oxytocin, and endorphins) and decrease the

Positive emotions increase the level of happy hormones (serotonin, dopamine, oxytocin, and endorphins) and decrease the level of stress hormones (adrenaline, cortisol, and norepinephrine).

level of stress hormones (adrenaline, cortisol, and norepinephrine). The second type of emotion is negative or unhealthy emotion, which leads to mental and emotional illness by causing stress and worry. Notice that every positive emotion has its negative counterpart. For example, hope is positive, while fear is negative. Calmness is positive, while anger is negative. There is a wise Buddhist saying: "Holding on to anger is like drinking poison and expecting the other person to die."

Emotions like worry, stress, anxiety, fear, anger, guilt, sadness, disgust, etc., are the breeding ground for ill health. Not only that, but these emotions are also detrimental to your social well-being. Hence, learning to develop healthy emotions is one of the most important steps to optimal well-being. All emotions arise from our thoughts, so it is important to control our thoughts to keep a check on the emotions. For example, worry arises when someone is always living in the future, and, half of the time, things we worry about do not even happen. Worry is like a rocking chair. It will give you something to do but won't take you anywhere. One experiences guilt because they are living in the past and trying to change the past, which is not possible. You learn from it and grow. The best way to maintain healthy emotions is to live in the present.

> *"Yesterday is history. Tomorrow is a mystery.*
> *Today is a gift. That is why it is called*
> *the present."* — *Alice Morse Earle*

If we learn to control our thoughts, nothing can phase us even when the situation is not under our control. Outside situations should not control our emotions, but, instead, our emotional stability should empower us to overcome situations in life. There is a famous quote: "Tough times never last, but tough people do." When our emotional stability is independent of our situations, we will not be stressed and will be able to boost our wellness. Emotionally stable people can remain calm under pressure and respond to any situation instead of reacting to it. Our ability to stay calm and happy in any situation will give us the gift of emotional, mental, physical, and social wellness.

Here are a few tips on how to remain calm amidst chaos and develop healthy emotions:

- First and foremost, decide to train your mind to develop emotional stability. It's easier said than done, and it will require a lot of practice, discipline, as well as mindfulness. It will require you to mentally slow down and check your thoughts every now and then because your emotional stability will depend on the quality of your thoughts. Your thoughts become feelings. So, whenever you feel low or sad, check your thoughts. Your feelings will become actions, and your actions will become habits, and your habits will form your destiny. Thus, your thoughts and your words will become your world.

- Decide to protect your mind by controlling what you feed it. Your thoughts depend on what you put into your mind. Do you know the term GIGO? Garbage in, garbage out. We use the five senses to feed our minds. Touch, sight, smell, hearing, and taste. We must control what goes in through these five senses to protect our minds. For example, don't watch or listen to the news, or anything negative, in the morning or before going to bed. Also, you don't need to stay updated on the news every half hour. You will drastically cut down on the negative input by making this small change. Additionally, don't participate in gossip or backbiting.

- Breathe consciously. When any negative thought comes to your mind, you will realize it because you will start getting depressed, stressed, or anxious. So, be mindful of your feelings and track your thoughts when you are feeling low. Practice pranayama, or coherent breathing, as it might help you calm down and feel better.

- Switch your thoughts by focusing on your blessings. During any given day, it's likely that seven out of ten things go in our favor, but our environment has conditioned us to focus on what is going wrong. Practice an attitude of gratitude to switch your focus to optimism. Savor moments of joy. Be present in the now. When you are worried, chances are you are living in the future. When you are sad or depressed, chances are you are living in the past. It's okay to plan for the future and set goals, but live in the now. Also, it is okay to visit the past sometimes, to learn from our mistakes, but don't live there.

- Take time out for yourself. Practice self-care. It can be as simple as taking a bubble bath, going for a walk, exercising, watching a comedy, or listening to music. Take 20 to 30 minutes out of every day to do whatever makes you feel light and joyful. Self-care is an excellent way to lift your spirits. If you are seeking ideas for self-care that don't break the bank, visit _www.krutithakore.com/check-out-my-books_.

- Process your emotions. Don't suppress them, but also don't express them without processing and understanding them first. For example, there is no need to express your anger as soon as you feel angry with someone. Instead, take deep breaths, regain your emotional stability, and then process your emotions by asking yourself questions about what made you feel a certain way. This will give you the ability to handle any situation maturely.

- Listen to your body. If you are hungry, nourish it with good quality, nutritious food. If you are thirsty, drink good quality water, and if you are tired, take a break and rest. If you feel restless, go for a walk or exercise. A healthy body will give you the gift of a healthy mind and vice versa. Hunger or fatigue might make you angry or cranky.

- Journaling to release stress is a great idea. Journal all your thoughts and emotions. You can also write a gratitude journal to help you stay focused on your blessings. It can become difficult to write and maintain a gratitude journal because it is just one more task to do, but if you tend to naturally gravitate toward negativity, complaining, or finding faults, this habit will change your life. It will help you to shift your focus from negativity to positivity. So set aside 10 to 15 minutes before your bedtime and write five things you can be grateful about. It doesn't have to be deep or elaborate, or fancy. It can be as simple as "I am thankful for my family" or "I am thankful for my nourishing breakfast." You will be surprised to find several simple things to be thankful about with the slight shift in focus that comes from gratitude journaling, and you will also attract more and more good things into your life that you can be grateful about. Gratitude journaling is the best way to develop an attitude of gratitude. On the days when you are feeling down, you can visit your journal and read it repeatedly to shift your focus on positivity. Focusing on blessings is a sure-shot recipe to develop healthy emotions and reduce stress. Research shows that people who have a habit of gratitude journaling have a significant reduction in chronic inflammation. When we change our thoughts and attitude toward life in a positive manner, our bodies respond to it drastically, which results in physical, emotional, mental, and spiritual well-being.
- Utilize the S.T.O.P. method where S stands for Stop, T stands for take a deep breath, O stands for observe your feelings and

thoughts without judgment, and P stands for proceed to choose with love and compassion.

- Visualize a stop sign in your mind to calm down before lashing out.
- Take a deep breath and count to 10 before speaking when upset.
- Meditation, yoga, and pranayama. These are sure-shot methods to calm an overactive mind.
- It is said that your eyes are the gateway to your soul. Sight is the best way to heal the soul and mind. Activities like spending time in nature, developing a hobby like gardening, going for a hike, going to a park for a jog, or doing yoga on a beach while enjoying sunrise can help you stay grounded, release happy hormones, and develop emotional well-being.
- According to Ayurveda, dosha imbalance in the mind can cause emotional turbulence. The imbalance of doshas on a mental level can be balanced by sound, sight, and smell. The use of aromatherapy and essential oils is beneficial. The scent of camphor, clove, and eucalyptus can remove the sluggishness and lethargy. At the same time, the cooling, flowery fragrance of jasmine, sandalwood, and rose can help reduce anger and resentment from an out-of-balance pitta mind. Lavender and chamomile fragrances can help reduce anxiety and worry.
- Music has remarkable healing properties. Sounds of flute or ocean waves can calm your mind and remove anxiety, while energetic sounds, like samba, can remove lethargy and sluggishness. Mantras also have excellent healing properties. Just sitting quietly and meditating at the sound of Om will help you heal your emotions.
- Learn the art of conscious communication. Conscious Communication is a skill, not a talent, and, hence, it can

be acquired if we try to learn it. Conscious communication is our ability to communicate with ourselves clearly and compassionately, as well as with others. It is our ability to think wisely and stop that nonstop chatter that goes on in our minds. It is our ability to remove the negative self-talk and whining from our vocabulary, which makes us feel like a victim and hurts our self-esteem. Our emotional well-being depends on how we communicate with ourselves, as well as with others.

> *Conscious communication is our ability to communicate with ourselves clearly and compassionately, as well as with others.*

Conscious communication teaches us to respond calmly to any person or situation like a mature adult instead of reacting. Once we acquire this skill, it not only reduces stress and improves our emotional well-being, but it also enhances our social well-being and improves our relationships.

In brief, here is the five-step process to improve Conscious Communication, which I learned when I was studying to become a perfect health Ayurvedic lifestyle instructor at The Chopra Center:

Step 1: What Happened?

When something goes wrong, take a few deep breaths. It will help you calm down. Then, mentally review the whole situation as a neutral third person and ask yourself, "What happened?" Count to 10 if needed so that you can gain emotional stability. Come to the Present Moment. If this event reminds you of an unpleasant past, just taking a few deep breaths and counting to 10 will help you come back to the present moment. Stay grounded. Looking out a window at nature is a great way to calm down. Close your eyes and tell yourself that whatever happened before was in the past and not the present. This situation is not a repetition of the past. Describe the Facts of the Situation from the Third Party's Point of View. Give as many details as possible and identify triggers. Also, don't judge yourself or anyone else. Keep a neutral perspective. Develop a pure and non-biased heart.

Step 2: How am I Feeling?

Describe your feelings, choosing words that describe your core emotions instead of words that reinforce feelings of victimization. Avoid words like cheated, abandoned, betrayed, manipulated, used, unappreciated, let down, overworked, unwanted, etc.

Step 3: What Do I Need That I'm Not Receiving?

The four fundamental human needs, which we all want are attention, affection, acceptance, and appreciation. Introspect and find out what you are not receiving.

Step 4: What am I Asking For?

Identify the specific behaviors or actions that would fulfill your needs. At the same time, understand that the person you are dealing with is not perfect. They might be able to fulfill your needs or might not be able to fulfill them. Hence, it is important to surrender to the uncertainty, allow yourself to be vulnerable, and ask for what you need. Observe the response of the other person from a state of calm awareness.

Step 5: What is the Gift or Opportunity in this Situation?

No matter how the situation unfolds, it's important to look deeply at the experience and what we learned. The person you are dealing with may understand your point of view and might be able to meet your expectations. This will be a win-win situation. It is a "glow" moment. In case this is not possible, and they do not understand your point of view or cannot meet your expectations, you can use the journaling technique and list what you learned from this situation.

This will be your "grow" moment. Either way, it will be a great experience, as you will either win or grow.

Finally, it is essential to develop self-love. Here is the list of daily self-check questions to focus on self-love:

- Am I getting enough rest?
- How am I feeling today?
- Am I always uplifting myself?
- What am I doing for self-care and self-love?
- What am I grateful for?
- Am I nourishing myself with the right foods and the right experiences?
- Do I have a work-life balance?

References:

- *Chopra, D. D., Kshirsagar, D. S., Simon, D. D., Patel, D. S., Porter, D. V., Saint, D. M., Gabriel, R., Stern, E., & Nadarajah, M. (2019, November). The perfect health ayurvedic lifestyle online enrichment program. Session 1 - 15.*
- *Fredrickson, B. L., Boulton, A. J., Firestine, A. M., Van Cappellen, P., Algoe, S. B., Brantley, M. M., Kim, S. L., Brantley, J., & Salzberg, S. (2017). Positive Emotion Correlates of Meditation Practice: A Comparison of Mindfulness Meditation and Loving-kindness Meditation. Mindfulness, 8(6), 1623–1633. https://pubmed.ncbi.nlm.nih.gov/29201247/*
- *Fredrickson B. L. (2001). The role of positive emotions in positive psychology. The broaden-and-build theory of positive emotions. The American psychologist, 56(3), 218–226. Available from: https://www.ncbi.nlm.nih.gov/pmc/articles/PMC3122271/*

CHAPTER 27

Step 9: Meditation

⟨⟨⟨⟨

"Meditation is like a gym in which you develop the powerful mental muscles of calm and insight." – Ajahn Brahm

Before we dive deep into the benefits of meditation, let us get into more details about what meditation is. In this super busy world, we all are highly active, both physically and mentally. Our lives are full of activities, and we take pride in calling ourselves "highly busy." Today's world is full of competition, and it is survival of the fittest. Humans are running in the rat race from morning to night just to get ahead. This results in stress, anxiety, fatigue, tension, and, eventually, burnout.

People use stimulants, like caffeine, just to feel energized. Over and above that, the use of smart devices, social media, TV, movies, and YouTube is increasing every day, so our brain never gets rest. Most humans do not get enough sleep, or the quality of their sleep is very poor, so they wake up tired. Their day starts with caffeine. Tired brains and tired bodies impact the quality of life by reducing productivity, decreasing health, and negatively affecting relationships.

So, what is the solution? There are several answers to this question, like technology detox, improving the quality of sleep, eating a balanced diet, managing priorities, learning proper time-management skills, self-love, taking time out to wind down at night, and taking time to recharge, but meditation is the most effective way to reduce stress, anxiety, fatigue so that you can attain emotional and mental well-being. Hence, it is vital, and it tops the list.

What is Meditation and What is it Not?

Numerous studies are being conducted regarding the correlation between meditation and mental, as well as physical health, and the results are fascinating. Data shows that meditation has impressive neurological and physical benefits. Meditation is a method to quiet the mind. It is a way to recharge or to slow down so that we can speed up. Meditation is the journey from noise to silence. It allows us to quiet the noise of our minds to become more aware and present. Some people assume that meditation is tied

Conscious communication is our ability to communicate with ourselves clearly and compassionately, as well as with others.

Meditation is a process that helps us go within to gain knowledge about who we really are, what our purpose is and opens the door to infinite possibilities.

to a religion or culture. That is not true. Meditation has nothing to do with any religion or culture. Meditation is for everyone and has no boundaries. Meditation is a process that helps us go within to gain knowledge about who we really are, what our purpose is and opens the door to infinite possibilities.

Here are the benefits of meditation:

- Meditation is a great tool to improve the quality of our life.
- Meditation improves health, both physical and emotional. When we are stressed, we snap at people and react to any situation which makes us feel uncomfortable. Meditation teaches us to respond to situations instead of reacting to them. Thus, meditation improves relationships.
- Meditation improves physical health by decreasing inflammation, lowering blood pressure, strengthening our immune system, and reducing autoimmune diseases.
- Meditation turns off genes responsible for diseases like diabetes, Alzheimer's, some types of cancer, and autoimmune diseases.
- Meditation reduces age-related memory loss.
- Meditation turns on the genes responsible for good health.
- Meditation slows down the aging process by increasing levels of the enzyme telomerase.
- Meditation increases the production of hormones like serotonin, oxytocin, endorphins, and dopamine. Thus, it helps increase joy, happiness, peace, love, compassion, relaxation, and gratitude.
- Meditation decreases stress hormones like cortisol and adrenaline. Thus, meditation reduces stress, fatigue, anxiety, and burnout.
- Meditation activates our parasympathetic nervous system and helps improve digestion, heart health, and GI health.

- Meditation increases the production of the anti-aging hormone DHEA and human growth hormone (HGH).
- Meditation increases mental sharpness, attention span, focus, and memory. Thus, it improves our ability to learn new things. Meditation is an excellent way for students to improve their grades. It also enhances our productivity at work and indirectly enhances our financial well-being.
- Meditation helps one cultivate positive emotions and loving-kindness toward oneself and others, improving emotional and social well-being.
- Last but not least, meditation improves our creativity and opens doors to unlimited possibilities. Meditation helps quiet our minds. Just observe the waves when we are at the beach. The waves crashing on the shore are very turbulent, with lots of activity going on at the surface. We will never find pearls at the surface of the ocean due to the hyperactivity and turbulence, but when we dive deep into the ocean, the water is still. Almost zero turbulence. That's where we find the precious pearls. The same is true for our minds. Pearls of wisdom are found when our mind is quiet.

When we throw a stone into turbulent water, nothing happens. But, if we throw a stone into quiet water, it creates ripples. The same is true when an idea comes to a busy mind: Nothing happens when there is a lot of noise. Before we can implement it, our mind starts thinking about something else. But, when an idea comes to a quiet mind, we can implement it and open doors to unlimited possibilities. Thus, meditation helps us reach our fullest potential.

This reminds me of a story. Once Buddha was walking from one town to another with a few of his followers. This was in the initial days. While they were traveling, they happened to pass a lake. They stopped there, and Buddha told one of his disciples, "I am thirsty. Do get me some water from that lake there."

The disciple walked up to the lake. When he reached it, he noticed that some people were washing clothes in the water and, right at that moment, a bullock cart started crossing through the lake. As a result, the water became very muddy, very turbid. The disciple thought, how can I give this muddy water to Buddha to drink? So, he came back and told Buddha, "The water in there is very muddy. I don't think it is fit to drink."

After about half an hour, again, Buddha asked the same disciple to go back to the lake and get him some water to drink. The disciple obediently went back to the lake. This time, he found that the lake had absolutely clear water in it. The mud had settled down, and the water above it looked fit to be had. So, he collected some water in a pot and brought it to Buddha.

Buddha looked at the water, and then he looked up at the disciple and said, "See what you did to make the water clean? You let it be— and the mud settled down on its own, and you got clear water. Your mind is also like that. When it is disturbed, just let it be. Give it a little time. It will settle down on its own. You don't have to put any effort to calm it down. It will calm down effortlessly."

What did Buddha emphasize here? He said, having "peace of mind" is not a strenuous job; it is an effortless process. When there is peace inside you, that peace permeates to the outside. It spreads around you and in the environment, such that people around you start feeling that peace and grace.

There are several types of meditation practices. The most popular ones are the following:

- Mindfulness meditation
- Spiritual meditation
- Focused meditation
- Movement meditation
- Mantra meditation
- Transcendental meditation
- Progressive relaxation
- Loving-kindness meditation
- Visualization meditation
- Rajyoga meditation
- Yoga meditation or yoga nidra.

Not all meditation practices are for everyone, but you can always learn more about these and figure out what works best for you. Once you find the right one, stick to it.

References:

- *Chopra, D. D., Kshirsagar, D. S., Simon, D. D., Patel, D. S., Porter, D. V., Saint, D. M., Gabriel, R., Stern, E., & Nadarajah, M. (2019, November). The perfect health ayurvedic lifestyle online enrichment program. Session 1–15.*
- *Norris, C. J., Creem, D., Hendler, R., & Kober, H. (2018). Brief Mindfulness Meditation Improves Attention in Novices: Evidence From ERPs and Moderation by Neuroticism. Frontiers in human neuroscience, 12, 315. https://www.ncbi.nlm.nih.gov/pmc/articles/PMC6088366/*

- *U.S. Department of Health and Human Services. (n.d.). Meditation: In-depth. National Center for Complementary and Integrative Health. Retrieved December 2, 2021, from https://www.nccih.nih.gov/health/meditation-in-depth.*
- *Fredrickson, B. L., Boulton, A. J., Firestine, A. M., Van Cappellen, P., Algoe, S. B., Brantley, M. M., Kim, S. L., Brantley, J., & Salzberg, S. (2017). Positive Emotion Correlates of Meditation Practice: A Comparison of Mindfulness Meditation and Loving-kindness Meditation. Mindfulness, 8(6), 1623–1633. https://pubmed.ncbi.nlm.nih.gov/29201247/*

CHAPTER 28

Step 10:
Pranayama and
Intentional Breathing

⫣⫣⫣

When the breath wanders, the mind wanders.
But when the breath is steady, the mind too
will be steady,
and the yogi will achieve long life.
Therefore one should learn to regulate
the breath. – Hatha Yoga Pradapika

Pranayama, which is an integral part of yoga, is a practice to become mindful of the breath, which helps improve physical, emotional, and spiritual health. Pranayama is a Sanskrit word made of two Sanskrit words, prana (vital life force) and ayama (to control or expand). Pranayama helps improve and strengthen the communication between mind and body. It is an excellent way to enhance physical and emotional health.

Pranayama breathing techniques are part of the ancient Indian yogic tradition, and it is said that it came into existence, along with yoga, meditation, and Ayurveda, around 5000 BC. Yoga, pranayama, and meditation are also part of Ayurvedic practices. They are recorded within ancient texts like Vedas and the yoga sutras, and these texts mention pranayama as a foundational aspect of yoga practice.

Benefits of Pranayama

- Pranayama helps us to control our minds and our thoughts. It activates the parasympathetic nervous system, which is responsible for rest and digestion, promoting healing and rejuvenation.
- Several research studies show that, by practicing pranayama regularly, one can:
  - Reduce anxiety and depression.
  - Stabilize blood pressure.
  - Improve sleep.
  - Reduce stress.
  - Increase energy levels and mental focus, as well as performance.
  - Enhance the capacity of the lungs. I believe that pranayama is a detox for the lungs.
  - Reduce PTSD.
  - Improve cardiovascular health.
- Enhances cognitive performances.

Pranayama helps us to control our minds and our thoughts. It activates the parasympathetic nervous system, which is responsible for rest and digestion, promoting healing and rejuvenation.

- Reduces cravings for cigarettes.
- Many studies have documented the beneficial effects of pranayama on COPD and asthma.

Here are some simple pranayama techniques and their benefits. You can learn them from a qualified professional or yoga teacher.

1. **Coherence Breathing:** Coherence breathing offers many healing benefits, including decreased anxiety and depression, improved sleep, strengthened immune function, reduced inflammation, and increased resilience. This practice is suitable for all doshas.
2. **Nadi Shodhana (Alternate Nostril Breathing):** Nadi means the channel of circulation, and shodhana means cleansing. This pranayama helps remove emotional blockages, calm the mind, reduce anxiety stress, and improve sleep.
3. **Ujjayi (The Oceans Breathe):** Ujjayi can energize the body, calm down the mind by releasing feelings of irritation, and stabilize the cardiorespiratory system. It is beneficial for all the doshas, and people with aggravated pitta dosha can significantly benefit from it because of its cooling effect.
4. **Kapalbhati:** In Sanskrit, Kapal means forehead, and bhati means shining. Practicing kapalbhati regularly leads to a shining face with an inner radiance. It is highly energizing pranayama that helps improve digestion and cleanses the respiratory system. It is not recommended for pregnant women or people with heart disease, high blood pressure, hernia, or certain other medical conditions.
5. **Bhramari (Humming Bee Breath):** This is very calming pranayama. It helps to activate the parasympathetic nervous system and puts the body in rest-and-restore mode. It improves

concentration, reduces stress, relieves tension and anxiety. It soothes the nerves and releases cerebral tension.

A verse in the Sama Veda cautions, "Yatha sinho gaja vyadho, bhavedvashya shanaiha. Thartheva sevitho vayurnyartha hanthi sadhakam" ("Just like an elephant, a lion or a tiger can be tamed slowly and gradually, in the same way, a practitioner should try to tame their breath slowly, or else it kills the practitioner themselves").

As a beginner, it is very important that you don't start performing complex pranayama practices without learning them properly. First and foremost, learn to be mindful about your breath and just learn basic deep breathing techniques. Learn how to inhale (purak), how to hold your breath for five seconds or less (kumbhak), how to exhale (rechak), and how to hold it again for five seconds or less (shunyak). First, get used to these four basic steps. Then pranayama should be done very calmly, in a meditative sitting position. The spine should be straight, and the mind should be calm. It is essential to learn how to do pranayama properly from a professional before performing it on your own. If you are not able to learn pranayama, just taking a few deep breaths from the belly while mentally staying focused on the breath and exhaling will also be highly beneficial.

A verse in the Sama Veda cautions, "Yatha sinho gaja vyadho, bhavedvashya shanaiha. Thartheva sevitho vayurnyartha hanthi sadhakam" ("Just like an elephant, a lion or a tiger can be tamed slowly and gradually, in the same way, a practitioner should try to tame their breath slowly, or else it kills the practitioner themselves").

References:

- *Sharma, V. K., Trakroo, M., Subramaniam, V., Rajajeyakumar, M., Bhavanani, A. B., & Sahai, A. (2013). Effect of fast and slow pranayama on perceived stress and cardiovascular parameters in young health-care students. International journal of yoga, 6(2), 104–110. https://pubmed.ncbi.nlm.nih.gov/23930028/*
- *Pramanik T, Pudasaini B, Prajapati R. Immediate effect of a slow pace breathing exercise Bhramari pranayama on blood pressure and heart rate. Nepal Med Coll J. 2010 Sep;12(3):154-7. PMID: 21446363. Available from: https://pubmed.ncbi.nlm.nih.gov/21446363/*
- *Kuppusamy, M., Kamaldeen, D., Pitani, R., Amaldas, J., & Shanmugam, P. (2017). Effects of Bhramari Pranayama on health - A systematic review. Journal of traditional and complementary medicine, 8(1), 11–16. Available from: https://www.ncbi.nlm.nih.gov/pmc/articles/PMC5755957/*
- *Chopra, D. D., Kshirsagar, D. S., Simon, D. D., Patel, D. S., Porter, D. V., Saint, D. M., Gabriel, R., Stern, E., & Nadarajah, M. (2019, November). The perfect health ayurvedic lifestyle online enrichment program. Session 1–15.*
- *Dinesh, T., Gaur, G., Sharma, V., Madanmohan, T., Harichandra Kumar, K., & Bhavanani, A. (2015). Comparative effect of 12 weeks of slow and fast pranayama training on pulmonary function in young, healthy volunteers: A randomized controlled trial. International journal of yoga, 8(1), 22–26. https://www.ncbi.nlm.nih.gov/pmc/articles/PMC4278131/*
- *Kuppusamy, M., Kamaldeen, D., Pitani, R., & Amaldas, J. (2016). Immediate Effects of Bhramari Pranayama on Resting Cardiovascular Parameters in Healthy Adolescents. Journal of clinical and diagnostic research: JCDR, 10(5), CC17–CC19. https://www.ncbi.nlm.nih.gov/pmc/articles/PMC4948385/*

CHAPTER 29

Step 11: Nurturing Relationships and Social Support

મિત્ર એવો શોધવો ઢાલ સરીખો હોય,
સુખમાં પાછળ પડી રહે, દુઃખ માં આગળ હોય.

Find a friend who is like an armor. Just like armor
shields a warrior in times of battle, a true friend
will stand by your side in tough times.

We, humans, are social animals, and our social well-being plays an essential role in our optimal well-being. Spend some quality time with your loved ones. Fill up your emotional cup. We all need to be loved and give love. To love someone unconditionally, we need to first accept them as they are, and the same is true for self-love; hence it's vital that we develop unconditional acceptance and love towards ourselves and others. We have a need to stay connected with people. As you may have observed, during the COVID pandemic, when we all had to follow social distancing rules, after a while, people were burned out. Thank God for social media, as we could stay socially connected while maintaining social distance.

Social well-being means how well you are able to maintain your relationships with your loved ones and friends, how well you interact with society, and your ability to give back selflessly.

Social well-being means how well you are able to maintain your relationships with your loved ones and friends, how well you interact with society, and your ability to give back selflessly. This could mean giving back to your community or to a worthwhile cause.

Here are some tips on how to improve your relationships and social well-being:

- Giving back to society is one of the best ways to improve your optimal well-being. You don't have to be wealthy to give, as you can give your time and services. Just be open to the idea of adding value to others, and you will be surprised how much difference you can make. If you are busy and don't have a lot of time to give, just give a sincere compliment or give a smile or show genuine care. There are several benefits of giving and volunteering, like improved mood, improved self-esteem, increased happiness, fostering relationships, and increased ability to make new friends.
- Tell your near and dear ones how much you love them. Let

go of ego. You can either be right or be rich in relations as, wounds caused by words take a long time to heal. Choose your words wisely. Join a book club or attend meetups with like-minded people and build new friendships. Choose the right company. In Sanskrit, there are two words, "Sangha" and "Satsang". Sangha means a community of like-minded people and Satsang means being in the company of people who share good values like honesty, truth, integrity, kindness, love, etc. There is a saying that associate with dreamers if you want to catch a dream. In the same way, it is important to choose the right association so that you can thrive and become a better human being. Take short trips or weekend picnics with friends and family. Build loving memories and let go of grievances.

> *You can either be right or be rich in relations as, wounds caused by words take a long time to heal.*

- Be a giver, not a taker. There are two types of people. The first type is the *taker*. These people are constantly thinking about how others can help them. How can they personally benefit, sometimes at the cost of others? They believe that everyone owes them something. They have entitlement issues. Even if they give, they expect some favor in return. They keep the count. This is mainly because they have limiting beliefs and are insecure within themselves.

- The second type is the *giver*. These people are constantly thinking about how they can add value to others and help others. Sometimes they even go out of their way to help others. They give just because they are givers and not because they have hidden agendas. They don't keep count. When they are helping others, they don't feel that the other person "owes them one." Be a cheerleader. Celebrate the success of other people. Don't be jealous. Jealousy is a limiting belief and comes from a place of insecurity. Be a cheerleader of people. Genuinely praise others for their qualities. No fake praises. Be authentic in your words and actions. You can be authentic in your praise if you are a keen observer. If you observe people, you will find a quality or two in them that you can praise. Whatever goes around comes back. Your time will come.

- Don't gossip. Gossip spreads negativity and ruins the culture of an organization or a family unit. We talked about detoxing in earlier chapters, and we are taking the concept of detox one step further in this chapter. Learn gossip detox as it plays an important role in enhancing your social well-being. If someone, tries to badmouth a person who is not present, refuse to participate in the conversation. You can gently inform them that you are on gossip detox. Keep in mind that people who will talk with you about someone else behind their back will talk about *you* behind your back.

- Be a fire extinguisher and not a flamethrower. In the event of any conflict, try to defuse the conflict instead of adding fuel to the fire. The best way to defuse conflict is to resolve it like a mature adult. Take a deep breath. Mentally step away. Look at the whole issue as an adult instead of as a child. Put the ego aside and reflect. Instead of blaming another person, first, decide whether you had any role to play in creating the conflict. Make another person feel safe by understanding their point of view. Put yourself in their shoes. Have a pure heart while resolving the conflict. If you did not have any role to play in creating the conflict, first figure out if the other person made a genuine mistake or whether they were deliberate.

Was the mistake due to a lack of skill or knowledge, or was it an attitude problem? Most conflicts happen due to a lack of communication. Help them understand the stakes and keep the end goal in mind.

- Last but not least, always go the extra mile. Do whatever it takes, plus some more, with an upbeat attitude, without complaining. Smile and have a can-do mindset.

Here's a short story I read a few years back that explains the meaning of deep nurturing relationships.

A monk was being interviewed by a journalist from New York.

Journalist: "Sir, in your last lecture, you told us about 'Contact' and 'Connection.' Can you elaborate on it?"

The monk smiled and asked the journalist: "Are you from New York?"

Journalist: "Yes."

Monk: "Who do you have in your immediate family?"

The journalist felt that the monk was trying to avoid his question. Yet the journalist said: "Mother expired. Father, three brothers, and sister."

The monk, with a smile on his face, asked again: "Do you talk to your father? When did you talk to him last?"

Journalist: "Maybe a month ago."

Monk: "Do your brothers and sisters meet often?"

With a sigh, the journalist said: "We met last at Christmas two years ago."

Monk: "How many days did you all stay together?"

Journalist: "Three days."

Monk: "How much time did you spend with your father? Did you ask how his days are passing after your mother's death?"

Drops of tears started to flow from the eyes of the journalist.

The monk said: "Don't be upset or sad. I am sorry if I have hurt you. But this is the answer to your question. You have *contact* with your family, but you don't have a *connection*. Connection is between heart and heart."

Journalist: "Thanks for teaching me an unforgettable lesson."

Don't maintain *contacts*. Remain *connected*.

References:

- *Harandi, T. F., Taghinasab, M. M., & Nayeri, T. D. (2017). The correlation of social support with mental health: A meta-analysis. Electronic physician, 9(9), 5212–5222. https://www.ncbi.nlm.nih.gov/pmc/articles/PMC5633215/*
- *Ozbay, F., Johnson, D. C., Dimoulas, E., Morgan, C. A., Charney, D., & Southwick, S. (2007). Social support and resilience to stress: from neurobiology to clinical practice. Psychiatry (Edgmont (Pa.: Township)), 4(5), 35–40. Available from: https://www.ncbi.nlm.nih.gov/pmc/articles/PMC2921311/*

CHAPTER 30

Step 12: Sound Financial Decisions (Peace of Mind)

"Money, like emotions, is something you must control to keep your life on the right track." — *Natasha Munson*

L ack of money is a top cause of stress for many. Several types of research have been done to understand the link between financial well-being and health. The psychological distress caused by financial stress may contribute to chronic acute-phase inflammation, resulting in anxiety, worry, depression, mood disorders, migraines, diabetes, sleep disorders, cardiovascular problems, high blood pressure. Financial stress may have an adverse impact on emotional, as well as physical, well-being.

When I am talking about health, I am not just addressing your physical health here. I am addressing all the aspects of overall well-being, including physical health, emotional and mental well-being, environmental well-being, social well-being, relationships, productivity, and purpose. Imagine your life as a wheel of a bicycle, and all these above-mentioned dimensions of overall well-being are the spokes of the wheel. Now, you see how they are interconnected? If one spoke is weak or broken, it has an adverse effect on all the other spokes.

Lack of money is one of the biggest causes of stress. Most divorces happen due to stress caused, either because of lack of money or lack of time for each other. It is well-known that people lose sleep due to financial stress. Quality of sleep impacts physical, mental, and emotional well-being. Emotional and mental well-being deteriorate due to stress and lack of sleep. People have mood swings, anxiety, and depression. It is like a vicious cycle. Stress reduces the quality of sleep, which in turn impacts health and creates more stress. Now you can see how financial well-being is related to emotional and mental health. Poor emotional and mental health reduces a person's ability to respond to life situations. People make mountains out of molehills just because they are stressed. Due to stress, people become angry, respond bitterly to minor day-to-day incidents, snap at others, become over-reactive, or dwell in self-pity. This is a sure-shot formula for creating a rift in any relationship. Thus, financial well-being also impacts your social well-being and relationships. Hence, financial stress is one of the major causes of high divorce rates.

Now, when you lack social support, your ability to bounce back from stress, anxiety, depression, etc., is decreased. People end up having addictions to alcohol, junk food, sugar, and other harmful substances just because of stress and anxiety. They make poor choices and errors in judgments. Their ability to discern right from wrong fades away. Also, due to lack of money, people may take two or three jobs just to stay afloat. This leads to a lack of time. You cannot pay attention to your physical health and relationships when you don't have time. You cannot take time out or spend money on self-care to exercise, eat healthy meals, or meditate when doing two or three jobs. You obviously will not get enough sleep in this situation, so everything goes downhill, and you feel stuck in a rut. All this drama in your life also affects your self-esteem and productivity. Now you see how a lack of financial discipline can become a disaster in all other areas of your life.

Like it or not, money (or lack of it) will influence many life decisions: where you live, what you eat, which school or universities your children would go to, how much time you will have for your family, etc. Thus, your socio-economic situation will control the quality of your life and your future generations. Financial burden, and the stress caused by it, also impact the well-being of children in the family. Research shows that when the family experiences overwhelming debt or financial burden, the stress not only impacts the health of adults in the family but also has a devastating impact on the well-being of the children in the family. School psychologists and guidance counselors have reported that the performance of children in schools is decreased and that children struggle to cope with the stress when their families suffer from financial problems.

Your socio-economic situation will control the quality of your life and your future generations.

Anything can be improved if you put your mind to it. The same is true for financial health. You must plan properly and be disciplined about delayed gratification. Stop money, time, and resources leaks. Seek the help of a professional if required.

Here are a few tips on how to improve your financial health:

- Track your financial well-being by visiting https://www.consumerfinance.gov/consumer-tools/financial-well-being/
- Be mindful about all sources of income and where your money is going. Then create a budget so that the expenses are less than the income.
- There are several ways to reduce expenses. Figure out what works for you.
- Pay yourself first by saving for the rainy day. Develop the habit of mandatory savings. Start small and increase your habit of savings.

> *Track your financial well-being by visiting https://www.consumerfinance.gov/consumer-tools/financial-well-being/*

- Stop eating out and start cooking at home.
- Cut out Netflix, cable, expensive hobbies and other unnecessary expenses. It will save both time and money.
- You don't have to buy the latest iPhone or gadget, or anything you don't need, just to impress others with the money you don't have.
- Identify opportunities to create multiple income streams. Identify your strengths and passions. If needed, inquire with your social circle or a mentor, and they may be able to shed some light on your strengths. Find opportunities to use your strengths to serve others in a way that can create income for you. For example, if you love pets, you could have a pet-sitting business on the side to generate extra income.
- You can also increase your income by switching to a higher-paying job. Invest in yourself, improve your skills and

self-esteem. Read self-help and self-development books like *The Magic of Thinking Big* by David J. Schwartz or *Think and Grow Rich* by Napoleon Hill. Your income depends on your self-esteem.

- Start paying off your credit cards. Start with a card with the highest interest rate first. See if debt consolidation makes sense for your situation.

- Stop impulse purchases. Most people go into debt to impress people they don't like, buying stuff they don't need with money they don't have. Develop the habit of paying with cash. Seeing the money leaving your pocket will help you realize the value of money and be more aware of your spending habits. Also, it will help you stay away from credit card debt.

- No more happy hours in the bar. It will save money, time, health, and relationships.

- Put all your cards in a safe and do not use them, no matter what. When making any purchases, pay with cash instead of a credit card. This habit will stop you from spending money you don't have.

- Automate your savings through payroll deductions. Maximize your 401k, IRAs, and HSAs.

- Use your tax refund for savings or for paying off your debt.

- Create emergency funds for a rainy day. Use your savings only for emergencies. Set some ground rules to spend this money only on real emergencies.

- Keep track of all due dates for your bills. Late fees can cause havoc on your budget.

- Find someone who has a high net worth. Seek out their help and see if they are willing to mentor you. If they agree, be in their back pocket. Follow their guidance.

Self-discipline is required to achieve success in anything. In the beginning, forming new habits might be hard, but it is not impossible. Keep in mind, with your habits, you are also impacting your life and the lives of your future generation. You are teaching your children and the next generation with your example. You are impacting the next generation positively or negatively, so make wise choices and positively impact your kids and grandkids. Leave behind a legacy that your future generations will be proud of.

With that, we are almost at the end of this book, and you have the 12 keys to open the mystical lock of optimal well-being. I know it might be too much to take in. You might be unsure about your ability to make changes and stick to them, as change is never easy, but I assure you that it is worth the effort, and you can do it. Take the first step toward positive change on faith. Use the supermarket approach while implementing the recommendations from this book. Start with what resonates with you the most, and once you get comfortable with the change, work on the next habit. When you achieve success in changing one habit, it will automatically inspire you and lead you toward changing the next one. Slowly and steadily, before you know it, you will be heading toward optimal well-being through lifestyle changes. It will take time and effort, but the results you will achieve will be worth the work.

In short, start small. On the first of every month, make a list of three old habits to let go of that are not serving you well and replace them with three new habits, which will

On the first of every month, make a list of three old habits to let go of that are not serving you well and replace them with three new habits, which will help you progress toward your goal of achieving optimal well-being.

help you progress toward your goal of achieving optimal well-being. The key is to remain consistent and persistent. Remember that Rome was not built in a day; it was built every day. Even though we just learned 12 steps to optimal well-being, this book will not be complete without the last two chapters, as it is almost impossible to achieve optimal well-being without setting SMART goals and keeping stress at bay with lots of love and lots of laughter. In the next two chapters, you will learn to keep stress at bay and set SMART goals.

Reference:

- *Sturgeon, J. A., Arewasikporn, A., Okun, M. A., Davis, M. C., Ong, A. D., & Zautra, A. J. (2016). The Psychosocial Context of Financial Stress: Implications for Inflammation and Psychological Health. Psychosomatic medicine, 78(2), 134–143. https://www.ncbi.nlm.nih.gov/pmc/articles/PMC4738080/*

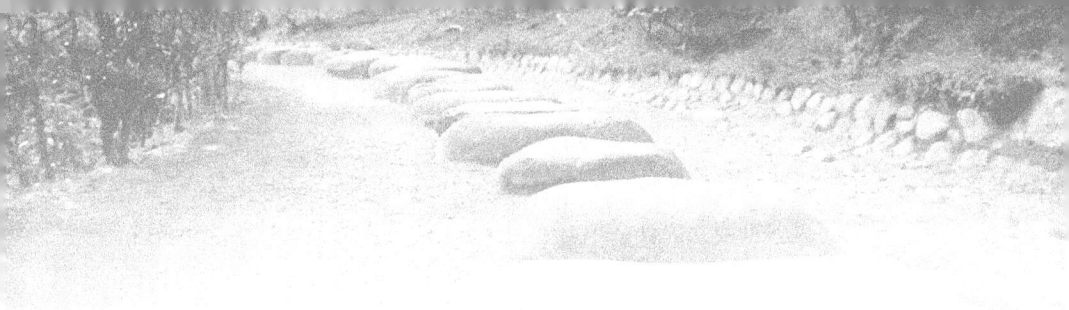

CHAPTER 31

Harmful Effects of Stress and Keeping Stress at Bay with Plenty of LOL (Lots of Love, Lots of Laughter)

If you are depressed, you are living in the past.
If you are anxious, you are living in the future.
If you are at peace, you are living in the present.
— *Lao Tzu*

Several studies in functional medicine/lifestyle medicine have proven that spirit, mind, and body are a whole unit and that they are interconnected. Hence, it is important to achieve spiritual well-being, emotional and mental well-being, and physical well-being to achieve optimal well-being. The emotional and mental disturbance will manifest as an illness in the body, and stress plays a major role in creating emotional and mental disturbance/illness.

What is stress? Stress is how your mind and body respond to life challenges, demands of life, trauma, or changes in your life. In short, how do you respond to anything unpleasant or outside of your comfort zone?

One must understand that life will always have challenges and obstacles. Not everything in life goes as we plan, and not everyone in our life behaves the way we want them to. Hence, no one can claim that their life is perfect or exactly the way they want it to be. So, it is important to learn to respond or cope in a healthy manner to challenges that life throws at us.

Stress is how your mind and body respond to life challenges, demands of life, trauma, or changes in your life.

How many times have you come across people who are happy under all circumstances? They might have endured severe trauma or job loss, but they have mastered their emotions. On the other hand, some people make a mountain out of a molehill. This doesn't mean that you have to bottle up all your emotions and you have lost the right to express them, but at the same time, when you experience any negative emotion, like anger, worry, guilt, anxiety, sadness, loneliness, fear, disgust, rage, or annoyance, be mindful about your emotions and learn healthy ways to cope with them before they get out of hand.

Everyone experiences stress in their life from time to time. Stress can be triggered by a one-time situation or can happen again and again. Several situations in life can be stressful. The most common triggers of stress are work or school pressure or family responsibilities. Also, stress can be triggered due to major loss, like loss of a job, loss of income, loss of a loved one, divorce, loss of a business, illness in the family, or personal illness. Over and above this, severe stress can occur due to traumatic events in life, like a major accident, war, assault, natural disaster, pandemic, etc. We also must understand that not all stress is bad because when you are in real danger, stress will prepare your body to face the danger or flee from it. In such situations, our survival depends on stress and how we respond to it. Sometimes stress can motivate people to work harder, especially in non-life-threatening situations, such as an interview for a new job or preparing for exams. But these situations are temporary, and stress-related to these situations is also temporary.

Problems happen when stress is not temporary. This kind of stress is widespread among one category of people, who always live in fear and anxiety, and most of the time, things they are worried or fearful about are not even true. People who are worried or fearful have constant "what if" thoughts going in their minds. For example, what if I lose my job? Or what if I met with an accident? They imagine the worst happening to them in the future and ruin their present with worry or fear.

Fear or worry is like a stationary bike. It takes up a lot of your mental energy but does not take you anywhere in life.

Fear or worry is like a stationary bike. It takes up a lot of your mental energy but does not take you anywhere in life. This doesn't mean that all fears are unnecessary, but the majority of them are imaginary. People who worry a lot, or are fearful, are living in the future, while people who are guilty all the time are living in the past. You cannot change your past, nor can you control your future, but you can surely control your present actions, which will determine your future. Additionally, you cannot control what happens to you or how people treat you, but you can control how you respond to it and how you treat yourself.

Long-term, chronic stress is a major cause of chronic inflammation. This can impact the immune system, digestion, cardiovascular health, sleep, and reproductive system. It can cause headaches, migraines, sadness, sleeplessness, anxiety, anger, and irritability, which can impact your performance at work or your relationships.

If you don't learn to cope with stress healthily, it can have a negative impact, not only on your physical well-being and emotional well-being but also on your relationships and social well-being, productivity at work, professional well-being, and financial well-being. Thus, stress, when not handled well, can easily cause fatigue and burnout. Stress for a sustained period may contribute to serious health conditions like heart disease, high blood pressure, stroke, diabetes, and other physical illnesses, along with mental and emotional illnesses like depression and anxiety.

Long-term, chronic stress is a major cause of chronic inflammation. This can impact the immune system, digestion, cardiovascular health, sleep, and reproductive system. It can cause headaches, migraines, sadness, sleeplessness, anxiety, anger, and irritability, which can impact your performance at work or your relationships.

As we now know how stress is created and what the harmful effects of stress are, there are several ways to keep stress at bay and reduce the negative effects of stress. The 12 steps that we discussed in the earlier chapters of the book are very effective in managing stress and reducing chronic inflammation.

As a reminder:

- Be mindful about your feelings and understand the signs your body shows in response to stress, such as difficulty sleeping, reduced appetite, irritability, worry, anger, low energy, and increased alcohol and other substance use.
- Be mindful of your thoughts. Think before you think. When you are conscious about your thoughts, you will learn to catch yourself when you are having negative thoughts of worry or fear. You will also catch yourself when you are living in the past and having guilt. Learn to replace these thoughts with positive thoughts. Replace fear with faith. Replace hate with love. Replace anger with forgiveness. Your emotions depend on your thoughts. So, to change your emotions, you must be mindful of your thoughts and change your thoughts. It is not easy, but it will be worth all the effort. With practice, you will master your thoughts.
- Be mindful about what you put in your mind. Constantly watching negativity on TV or the news or social media will create negative thoughts in your mind. Most of the time, the media only reports negative news, like pandemics, earthquakes, war, murder, etc., and if you keep watching this, it will impact your emotional well-being. It is not the media's fault that they only report bad news. If we were to look at the bright side and think logically, we'd realize there are billions of people living on this planet, and if the media reported on everything great

happening with these billions of people, there would be an infinite amount of news to publish. Compared to that reality (that bad news isn't happening for everyone everywhere), it is easy to report the bad news because bad news is limited. We just need to switch our thought processes. As Dr. Wayne Dyer once said, "When you change the way you look at things, the things you look at change."

- Method of conscious communication, which we discussed in Chapter 26, "Healthy Emotions," is another way to control your negative thoughts and emotions.

- Strive to have a proper work-life balance and try not to bring the stress of work home with you. Leave the bag of work-related stress at the front door of your home before you enter so that you can unwind, rejuvenate, and spend some quality time with your family.

- Exercise regularly, as just 30 minutes per day of exercise can improve your health and boost your mood.

- Meditation, breathing exercises, muscle relaxation, massage, bubble baths, spending quality time with people you love and cherish, spending time in nature, pursuing a hobby, getting a good night's sleep, staying hydrated, and eating well-balanced, nutritious meals are other ways to manage stress and show self-love.

- Laughter is the best medicine. In India, we have laughter clubs that promote and teach voluntary laughing. It is a form of yoga where practitioners will voluntarily burst in laughing without any reason because studies have proven that laughter is the fastest way to rebound from any negative emotions and balance your mind and body. A hearty laugh and good humor will draw people together, trigger healthy physical and emotional reactions in your body, strengthen your immune system, boost mood, reduce pain, and protect you from the negative effects of stress. Laughter reduces burdens, spreads joy and hope, improves relationships, and releases anger.

- Try a relaxing activity. Explore relaxation or wellness programs, which may incorporate meditation, muscle relaxation, or breathing exercises. Schedule regular times for these and other healthy and relaxing activities.

- Set goals and priorities. Decide what must get done now and what can wait. Do not bite off more than you can chew, or else you will choke. You do not have to be a people pleaser. It is okay to say "no" to new tasks if you start to feel like you're taking on too much. Try to be mindful of what you have accomplished at the end of the day, not what you have been unable to do.

- Use self-talk and affirmations to boost your mood. There are some great books on this topic, like *What to Say When You Talk to Yourself* by Dr. Shad Helmstetter. Talk to yourself to reassure yourself, so that you can calm yourself down. Just be sure that you remain positive, self-affirming, and constructive.

- Maintain a gratitude journal. The habit of counting your blessings can quickly shift your emotions to the positive side. Regularly keeping a gratitude journal can help you to stay hopeful during tough times. The purpose of gratitude journaling is to form a habit, and it takes 90 days to form a habit. Hence, I highly encourage you to use a gratitude journal consistently for the next 90 days till an attitude of gratitude is engraved in your psyche and becomes your second nature. To get started, check out my recently published gratitude journal with amazing motivational quotes by visiting *www.krutithakore.com/check-out-my-books*.

- Your social well-being plays an important role in your

emotional well-being. Stay connected with people you love and who love you. Surround yourself with your cheerleaders, who will uplift you and motivate you. Like everyone, you also might have a few people in your life who pull you down or demotivate you. It's vital for your emotional well-being and self-esteem that you dissociate from such people. If it is impossible to physically disassociate, develop a thick skin and mental fortitude so that their words and actions don't impact you. Stay connected with people who will believe in you, who make you feel happy, and provide support. Also, make sure that you can provide support for someone else who is in need. Don't be a taker, be a giver. People do not like to hang out with someone who is always complaining and whining. You also will have to try to be a cheerleader for other people.

- If stress is overwhelming, seek support. Verbalize and process your emotions by seeking professional help or help from friends, family members, or religious organizations.

- Talk to your health care provider or a health professional. Get proper health care for existing or new health problems. Effective treatments can help if your stress is affecting your relationships or ability to work.

- Most of the time, people are very compassionate toward others but hard on themselves. Show some compassion toward yourself. Cut yourself some slack. Practice self-love. Say no to self-criticism, self-doubt, and self-pity. Show plenty of self-love and self-respect toward your mind, spirit, and body. It is very easy to judge or criticize ourselves but this habit increases stress and dissatisfaction.

- Instead of focusing on weight loss and crash diets, one should always focus on feeling happy and healthy. If you love yourself, eating the right food, exercising, and taking care of yourself will be automatic, which will result in physical and emotional well-being. So, focus on health, not on appearance. The appearance will be the outcome of good health. Be very mindful of what you are thinking about your appearance when you look in the mirror. Consciously send the energy of appreciation to the body we already have. It is easier to cultivate love and respect for our bodies once we stop judging. Casual statements like "I am not happy about how I look" send a very powerful negative message to the mind and the body.

The truth is, how you look does not make you happy, but your happiness makes you look good. People around you may have opinions about how your body looks, but make sure that you don't criticize or reject your body. Take care of your body, keep it fit, but do it with the energy of love and appreciation. Allocate time and resources so that your body is clean, dressed comfortably, nourished properly, exercised adequately, and rested sufficiently. Get your

Casual statements like "I am not happy about how I look" send a very powerful negative message to the mind and the body.

daily dose of sunshine. At the same time, reduce or eliminate chemical pollutants in your environment, cosmetics, and cleaning products.

- Research shows that positive emotions suppress gene expressions that can lead to diseases, and they can lead to healthy gene expressions that are responsible for your well-being. Research has found a link between an upbeat mental state and improved health, including lower blood pressure, reduced risk for heart disease, healthier weight, better blood sugar levels, and longer life. Your state of mind affects your well-being, so choose positivity and happiness no matter what your situation is. Your situation should not affect your emotions, but your emotions will affect your situation. Happiness doesn't depend on how life treats us or on our possessions or social status, but on how we treat the situations in our life. It depends on our response and our attitude toward those situations. It comes from having a child-like faith in a higher power, knowing that no matter how bad the situation is

Research shows that positive emotions suppress gene expressions that can lead to diseases, and they can lead to healthy gene expressions that are responsible for your well-being.

today, this shall pass, and things will be better soon. "I am not happy because I am prosperous, but I am prosperous because I am happy." Our attitude attracts the right people and the right opportunities into our lives.

- Identify your purpose in life. Have a vision that is larger than life, and that requires faith and a positive mindset. A sense of higher purpose in life is the fuel for great health and longevity. In 2013, Barbara Fredrickson and colleagues conducted an experiment that has been repeated twice, and the results showed that people with no, or lower, life purpose had three impaired gene pathways in their immune systems, which compromised their immunity, whereas people with higher life purpose had healthy gene expression. In short, having a larger-than-life purpose can improve your immunity and well-being.

References:

- *U.S. Department of Health and Human Services. (n.d.). 5 Things You Should Know About Stress. National Institute of Mental Health. https://www.nimh.nih.gov/health/publications/stress/.*

- *Yim J. Therapeutic Benefits of Laughter in Mental Health: A Theoretical Review. Tohoku J Exp Med. 2016 Jul;239(3):243-9. doi: 10.1620/tjem.239.243. PMID: 27439375. https://pubmed.ncbi.nlm.nih.gov/27439375/*

- *Chopra, D. D., Kshirsagar, D. S., Simon, D. D., Patel, D. S., Porter, D. V., Saint, D. M., Gabriel, R., Stern, E., & Nadarajah, M. (2019, November). The perfect health ayurvedic lifestyle online enrichment program. Session 1–15.*

CHAPTER 32

Setting SMART Goals

⬰⬰⬰

*"If you don't strive for something worthwhile,
you will settle for anything."*

We are almost at the end of the book, and I understand it is a lot to take in. It's a new way of living life. The 12 steps that I have recommended for achieving optimal well-being are about lifestyle change. They are not a quick fix that you pursue temporarily and expect to achieve permanent goals. Change cannot happen overnight, and, even before a person starts working on changing their lifestyle, they go through weighing the pros and cons of the changes mentally. Similarly, you, too, might be mentally weighing the pros and cons of making a permanent lifestyle change. These stages of change are called pre-contemplation, contemplation, preparation, action, maintenance, and termination.

Precontemplation: In this stage, a person does not believe there is a problem or that change is required. Hence, there is no intention to change behavior in the foreseeable future. Most people in this stage are unaware of their problems or are in denial.

Contemplation: In this stage, people have started to realize that they need to change their lifestyles to achieve optimal well-being. At least there is the intention. They start weighing in the pros and cons of making changes. They intend to start changing their lifestyle for the better in the foreseeable future. They slowly start taking small steps toward making the lifestyle change. At the very least, they start believing that making the change can lead them to achieve a healthier life.

Change cannot happen overnight, and, even before a person starts working on changing their lifestyle, they go through weighing the pros and cons of the changes mentally.

Preparation: In this stage, people start putting actions behind their intentions. Individuals in this stage intend to take action soon or have started preparing to make changes. For example, this is the stage when people register for a gym membership or buy new gym clothes or throw out the junk food in their pantry. They start taking small baby steps toward making lifestyle changes.

Action: Action is the stage during which individuals modify their behavior and/or environment so that they can overcome the problems and achieve their goals, which, in this case, would be optimal well-being. At this stage, you should know that you may come across a few challenges or obstacles. Anticipate possible challenges and make a game plan for how to overcome them. Proper planning prevents poor performance. Invest in a coach and an accountability partner who will guide and inspire you to overcome the struggles and keep you moving forward.

Maintenance: In this stage, people have already changed their lifestyle habits and have sustained them for six months or so. They have already experienced the benefits because of the change they have made and are enjoying the rewards. They now intend to maintain their new lifestyle going forward so that they can enjoy the optimal well-being they have achieved.

Termination: In this stage, people have no desire to return to their unhealthy behaviors. They have no intention of going back to their old unhealthy lifestyle.

There are always chances of relapse at any stage, and, when that happens, be mindful and be gentle with yourself. Instead of going on a guilt trip or blaming the situation, just get back on track as soon as you realize that you need to up your game.

Making a huge change in one day might be very difficult but making small changes until you form a habit is attainable.

When I was growing up, my dad used to always remind me that life without a goal is like a ship without a radar. He would say, It's okay to miss your goal, but it is not okay to miss setting one.

Making a huge change in one day might be very difficult but making small changes until you form a habit is attainable. It is not easy to make long-term sustainable lifestyle changes, and, at the same time, it is important to set goals. When I was growing up, my dad used to always remind me that life without a goal is like a ship without a radar. He would say, It's okay to miss your goal, but it is not okay to miss setting one. For example, a basketball player should know where the basket is so that they can shoot. Similarly, you would not know what to shoot for without a goal. Hence, it is essential to set goals and then ensure that you hit every goal you set.

You should learn to set SMART goals that are specific, measurable, achievable/attainable, realistic/relevant, and time-bound.

Here are some details about setting SMART goals:

S – Set small goals. For example, I will replace one junk meal in a day with fruit or nuts. I will exercise 30 minutes a day instead of sitting on the couch and watching Netflix, and I will not watch TV until I complete the exercise.

M – Set measurable goals. Measure your progress. Maintain a diet diary and exercise diary. Use smart devices to log your activity and exercise. Use apps to record your diet. Decide to enter every single meal you eat into your diet diary.

A – Set attainable goals. Make sure you are physically capable of achieving your goal. Your goal should be a little bit out of your comfort zone so that it stretches you, but not so far out of your comfort zone that you fail on the first attempt. If you set an unrealistic goal, it will lead to stress, anxiety, and frustration. If you set goals that are too easy to achieve, you will get bored quickly. So, the key is to find a sweet spot and set a goal that will stretch you and promote growth. If you have never exercised before, do not set a goal to lift 100 pounds on day one.

R – Set realistic goals. Be realistic in setting goals. If it took you years to get into this situation, just changing your lifestyle for a day or a week, or a month will not be enough. Unrealistic expectations set you up for disappointments and failure.

T – Set time-bound goals. Set goals like: "I will wake up 30 minutes early on Mondays, Wednesdays, and Fridays to incorporate exercise into my schedule. I will test and record my blood sugar every morning before breakfast. I will incorporate fresh berries or dates into my breakfast instead of sugary donuts on the weekdays for the next 12 months. I will weigh myself and record my weight in the diary every Sunday morning before breakfast."

Now that you have learned the importance of SMART goals and how to set them, why don't you note down the steps you are going to take and your goals for achieving optimal well-being?

References:

- *Lacey, S. J., & Street, T. D. (2017). Measuring healthy behaviours using the stages of change model: an investigation into the physical activity and nutrition behaviours of Australian miners. BioPsychoSocial medicine, 11, 30. https://www.ncbi.nlm.nih.gov/pmc/articles/PMC5715498/*
- *Bailey R. R. (2017). Goal Setting and Action Planning for Health Behavior Change. American journal of lifestyle medicine, 13(6), 615–618. https://www.ncbi.nlm.nih.gov/pmc/articles/PMC6796229/*

CHAPTER 33

Conclusion

I hope that this book will inspire you to develop self-love so that you will devote more time and energy toward self-care. Most people do not understand the meaning of self-love. Self-love is not about taking a bubble bath or splurging on that expensive perfume or a candlelight dinner or getting into debt to buy that expensive car, but it is to be in a place where you are most comfortable, where you are at peace, and in a state of bliss. It is to strive for well-being in all dimensions of life so that you can live with ease and reach your fullest potential.

Self-love is choosing to love yourself unconditionally and to stay happy no matter what. Self-love is choosing to love yourself the way you are, despite your imperfections and weaknesses. Self-love is choosing to forgive yourself

Self-love is choosing to love yourself unconditionally and to stay happy no matter what. Self-love is choosing to love yourself the way you are, despite your imperfections and weaknesses.

for your mistakes and being willing to learn from those mistakes and start fresh. Self-love is choosing to nourish your body with the right nutrition and nourish your mind with the right books. Self-love is disassociating yourself from negativity and from people who pull you down while surrounding yourself with people who inspire you, believe in you, and cheer you up. Self-love is choosing to exercise, even when you feel like being a couch potato. Self-love is choosing to have self-control and choosing to have power over your addictions. Self-love is choosing meditation or exercise instead of going to happy hour. Self-love is above the superficial pleasures of life.

A person who loves themselves truly will always have power over their emotions and will always say no to harmful addictions. Make wise choices by thinking long-term and choose to say no to things that will give you unnecessary stress later. Fill up your cup with love so that you can pour love into the lives of others because you can only give what you have.

When you try to make any positive changes in your life, it is very natural to lose enthusiasm after a few days or at the sight of the slightest obstacle. That is the reason why gyms, which are packed in January of every year, lose half of the enthusiastic crowd by April. Most people break the resolutions they make on January 1st by January 15th. Research has shown that people who have a coach and an accountability buddy are more likely to pursue positive lifestyle changes even after the enthusiasm of the initial decision-making phase fades away. Hence,

Research has shown that people who have a coach and an accountability buddy are more likely to pursue positive lifestyle changes even after the enthusiasm of the initial decision-making phase fades away.

I recommend working with a coach who can be your accountability partner. A coach will help you to achieve a higher level of well-being and performance, in professional, as well as personal, life, when you feel it is hard to change those lifelong habits. By having a coach as your accountability partner, you can develop lifelong sustainable habits that will empower you to achieve optimal well-being.

To accomplish anything in life, it is important to determine your why, stay focused, and overcome obstacles. Coaching is the process that holds you accountable for making changes in your life and facilitates you to turn your dreams and goals into reality.

As experts correctly quote, your everyday habits become your destiny. Your coach is your accountability partner and your guide in this journey to excellence. With the help and encouragement from your coach, you will have self-motivation and self-regulation to form success habits so that you can embark upon a journey of change toward reaching your fullest potential. I invite you to join me in the movement: empowering one person at a time to improve the quality of their life and achieve optimal well-being.

References:

- *Perlman, A. I., & Abu Dabrh, A. M. (2020). Health and Wellness Coaching in Serving the Needs of Today's Patients: A Primer for Healthcare Professionals. Global advances in health and medicine, 9, 2164956120959274. https://doi.org/10.1177/2164956120959274*
- *May, C. S., & Russell, C. S. (2013). Health coaching: adding value in healthcare reform. Global advances in health and medicine, 2(3), 92–94. https://www.ncbi.nlm.nih.gov/pmc/articles/PMC3833544/*

- *Gordon, N. F., Salmon, R. D., Wright, B. S., Faircloth, G. C., Reid, K. S., & Gordon, T. L. (2016). Clinical Effectiveness of Lifestyle Health Coaching: Case Study of an Evidence-Based Program. American journal of lifestyle medicine, 11(2), 153–166. https://www.ncbi.nlm.nih.gov/pmc/articles/PMC6125027/*

www.ingramcontent.com/pod-product-compliance
Lightning Source LLC
Chambersburg PA
CBHW032051020426
42335CB00011B/288